SHAPING ACADEMIA FOR THE PUBLIC GOOD

Critical Reflections on the CHSRF/CIHR Chairs Program

Shaping Academia for the Public Good

Critical Reflections on the CHSRF/CIHR Chairs Program

EDITED BY LOUISE POTVIN &
PAT ARMSTRONG

UNIVERSITY OF TORONTO PRESS
Toronto Buffalo London

Toronto Buffalo London
www.utppublishing.com
Printed and bound by CPI Group (UK) Ltd, Croydon, CR0 4YY

ISBN 978-1-4426-4682-7

Library and Archives Canada Cataloguing in Publication

Shaping academia for the public good : critical reflections on the CHSRF/CIHR Chairs Program / edited by Louise Potvin & Pat Armstrong.

Includes bibliographical references and index.
ISBN 978-1-4426-4682-7 (bound)

1. Public health – Research – Canada. 2. Medicine – Research – Canada. 3. Education, Higher – Research – Canada. 4. Canadian Health Services Research Foundation. 5. Canadian Institutes of Health Research. 6. Research – Canada – Finance. 7. Federal aid to medical research – Canada. I. Armstrong, Pat, 1945–, editor of compilation II. Potvin, Louise, 1957–, editor of compilation

RA440.87.C3S53 2013 362.1′072071 C2013-902697-5

Canadian Foundation for Healthcare Improvement / Fondation canadienne pour l'amélioration des services de santé
CIHR IRSC Canadian Institutes of Health Research / Instituts de recherche en santé du Canada

This book was published with the support of the Canadian Foundation for Healthcare Improvement. The views expressed herein do not necessarily represent the views of the Government of Canada.
University of Toronto Press acknowledges the financial assistance to its publishing program of the Canada Council for the Arts and the Ontario Arts Council.

Canada Council for the Arts / Conseil des Arts du Canada
ONTARIO ARTS COUNCIL / CONSEIL DES ARTS DE L'ONTARIO
50 YEARS OF ONTARIO GOVERNMENT SUPPORT OF THE ARTS
50 ANS DE SOUTIEN DU GOUVERNEMENT DE L'ONTARIO AUX ARTS

University of Toronto Press acknowledges the financial support of the Government of Canada through the Canada Book Fund for its publishing activities.

Contents

Figures and Tables

Figures

Tables

Preface: The First Ones over the Barricade

Jonathan Lomas
Former Chief Executive Officer
Canadian Health Services Research Foundation

There is an old Swahili expression oft quoted by my public health colleague John Frank which, loosely translated, states: "The first ones over the barricade get a spear in the stomach." There were certainly times we felt the tip of cold steel at the Canadian Health Services Research Foundation (CHSRF) as we implemented the challenging idea that the task of educating the next generation of applied health services researchers might profit from collaboration and partnership between those in the health service and those in the academy. We were not the only ones, as the twelve chairs set many precedents in their home institutions and beyond as they developed their own innovative approaches to educating students and mentoring young faculty in the ways of applied research.

The chairs program was conceived in the late 1990s as part of a comprehensive applied training initiative – the Capacity for Applied and Developmental Research and Evaluation (CADRE) program – that also included regional training centres (see Martens et al., 2008), postdoctoral awards, and career renewal grants. Back then, universities and health sciences had (and, unfortunately, still have) a somewhat disparaging view of applied research and the social sciences. It is messy, often uncontrolled, unpredictable, and the very antithesis of the controlled, clean, and easily replicable laboratory experiments of the biomedical sciences or the prescribed routines of the clinical trial.

Ironically, this messiness demands greater creativity and elicits more intellectual engagement than the basic sciences. As a reviewer commented on one of my early career grant applications demanding a particularly complicated design: "Grinding rats is certainly easier than this health services research!" The research and training must have not only relevance to and resonance with the system it studies, but also methodological integrity in line with the standards of academic science. Applied health researchers are quintessentially Canadian – making something equally appealing and equally valid in the eyes of two communities with distinct values and preferences. The challenge, then, was not only to implement a new form of grant support that recognized this complexity in educating the next generation of applied researchers, but also to do so in an environment where there was little respect for such an endeavour and few models to follow.

How did I know that there was so little respect for the applied end of health services research? I came to lead CHSRF after fifteen years as a university-based applied health services researcher. I had experiences and anecdotes that significantly informed my view of the kind of new grant programming that was needed to enhance the reputation and role of applied health services research in universities. For instance, although I was a faculty member at McMaster University (arguably the most progressive of the health science centres in the country – hell, we even called ourselves a health sciences centre, not a medical school), I still found myself setting a begrudged precedent in the early 1990s when I won the right to supplement my academic letters of reference with ones from deputy ministers and others in the health system. One's impact on the health system clearly played a distant second fiddle to one's academic output and influence when it came to promotion and tenure in the university. (In 2003, CHSRF expanded a similar observation into a full-fledged study that demonstrated this was still the case) (Phaneuf et al., 2007).

Luckily, however, we were not alone. First, and most importantly, there was a renegade band of like-minded folks in appreciable numbers scattered around the country's universities and willing to apply to the chairs program. They may not yet have had respect, but they had idealism, energy, and a willingness to accompany us over that barricade in abundance. As you will read in the subsequent chapters, the chairs the reviewers selected may not have embarked on the journey had they known what was really in store for them, but none looks back now with regret.

Second, there were health service executives and senior bureaucrats in ministries of health interested in engaging themselves and their organizations with applied research and education. Not only did organizations like the Winnipeg Regional Health Authority or the Ontario and Quebec ministries of health help fund the chairs, but they and others such as the Montreal Regional Health Authority and the Nova Scotia Ministry of Health willingly released senior individuals to participate in the advisory committees, training, and research programs the incumbent chairs established.

Third, Health Canada encouraged the emerging Canadian Institutes of Health Research (CIHR) – only an interim entity as the chairs were launched – to co-fund CADRE as part of its flagship transition programs from the "old" Medical Research Council to the "new" form of federal granting council for health. This facilitated almost twice as many awards as originally planned and lent valuable credibility to the overall program. This partnership was significantly strengthened with the arrival of Morris Barer as the inaugural scientific director of CIHR's Institute of Health Services and Policy Research, who championed the program within the new organization.

Fourth, the nursing community had effectively lobbied the federal government for recognition of its value to research and CHSRF had received a $25-million, ten-year mandate to enhance nursing research capacity in Canada. Through the nursing advisory committee set up by CHSRF, the entire CADRE program and the chairs program in particular received strong support from the leaders of nursing administration and nursing research. It was within this context that either nurses or those with a nursing focus in their research and education received 50 per cent of the awarded chairs.

Finally, some universities, most notably the University of Montreal, caught a glimpse of the emerging "knowledge translation" era and saw the value of putting their own resources into a concerted effort to attract, support, and coordinate applications. There is no doubt that this effort was partly attributable to the excellent forerunner work of their provincial granting councils in both health (le Fonds de recherche santé du Québec) and social sciences (Conseil québécois de la recherche sociale), which alone among granting councils in the country had been encouraging academic networks embedded in health and social service systems for nearly a decade (Antil et al., 2003). Quebec was rewarded with fully 25 per cent of the awarded chairs (and subsequently received a regional training centre).

As stated earlier, the actual design of the chairs program leaned heavily on my own experience as a university-based health services researcher and the thoughts I had recently put down on how to improve the situation (Lomas, 1997). This was supplemented by the extensive granting experience of my director of research programs,

Linda Murphy, who had spent more than a decade on the other side of the fence disbursing funds through Health Canada's National Health Research and Development Program.

Four fundamental assumptions constituted the building blocks for the program:

1. We believed that increasing the amount of ongoing linkage and exchange between academics and system-based managers or policy makers would lead to their greater use of research. However, this was only likely to happen if the status and prestige of such applied work was raised in the university.
2. We needed to counteract the tradition of most prestigious personnel awards, which rewarded star researchers by alleviating them of formal teaching duties and ignoring their mentoring responsibilities; addressing the training shortfall would involve turning this tradition on its head.
3. We believed change would come from long-term support for innovative and energetic people and their imaginations, not from irregular grant funding of structures and projects.
4. We knew creating synergy between those engaged with the program (award holders and their students, program staff, and the partners) would multiply effectiveness and accelerate mutual learning.

Most of the specific design elements and rules of the chairs program can be traced back to these core assumptions. For instance, belief in the value of ongoing linkage and exchange with those in the system led us to require applicants to seek out decision-making partners. The need to improve the status of applied research in universities led us to set the award level as the most lucrative available at the time for national chairs, and the only ones to promise support that lasted a decade.[1] The failure of most other personnel awards to recognize the importance of teaching led us to give precedence to the education and mentoring activities of the chairs over their research. The need to identify the right people as chairs – the ones with enthusiasm, commitment, a track record in education, and at least ten more years of leadership in the academy – meant that we recruited international peer reviewers and hired head-hunters to do extensive reference checks on the short list. Finally, routine meetings of program participants once the initiative was underway helped all to do program adjustments and get mutual support and learning.

Almost immediately, two things stood out. First, there was an instant sense of a community united by a shared set of renegade ideas for bringing academic research and students into the health system. In that way, the program merely provided recognition and a home for the people who were already trying to bring reality to research or insert science into the system.

Second, these already busy applied academics were suddenly even busier. They had achieved success in their careers on their own merits and with a variety of largely haphazard accumulations of resources. The size and long-term security of the chairs program woke them all up to their greater potential as the head of a program. Their lives changed from those of university faculty members, albeit very successful and busy ones, to those of applied training program managers responsible for coordinating significant resources, research platforms, partnerships, and apprenticeships. Thus we, CHSRF, quickly uncovered the first of a number of miscalculations in our program design – we had not anticipated the extent of the administrative task we set for the chairs.

To their credit, the chairs rose willingly to this challenge, and over the initial years most found ways to use their resources to create administrative structures that unburdened them of the more mundane aspects of the task. It took them longer to convince us at CHSRF that we had underestimated the value of a vibrant research platform for their primary role of education and mentoring. Eventually they prevailed and we saw the light. They suffered largely silently as staff turnover at CHSRF sometimes delayed our responses or duplicated their work. Nevertheless, our semi-annual get-togethers in the early years gave chairs ample opportunity to give us feedback (an opportunity that was rarely foregone) and us a chance to make adjustments.

The fact that a community has emerged from the chairs program is evident in this book. As of the time of writing, the program has covered well over half its life and its community stretches well outside the number of chairs and partners. Countless students and junior faculty have been trained or mentored through their work, and numerous decision-makers in the health system have found value from their projects, placements, and exposure to evidence-informed decision-making. Other agencies – the Public Health Agency of Canada, for example – have subsequently copied its model. Innovations in education, mentoring, applied research methods, knowledge translation, partnership management, and so on will all be found in the pages that follow – pages that document the lived experience of being the first over the barricades. *Shaping Academia* is a testament to the innovation that can happen when you give a radical new mandate and secure resources to bright and imaginative people in the university.

NOTE

1 Unfortunately, we were quickly trumped on financial prestige with the federal government's announcement of the millennium Canada Research Chairs. Sometimes even the best-laid plans are just plain sideswiped.

REFERENCES

Antil, T., Desrochers, M., Joubert, P., & Bouchard, C. (2003). Implementation of an innovative grant programme to build partnerships between researchers, decision-makers and practitioners: The experience of the Quebec Social Research Council. *Journal of Health Services Research and Policy, 8*(suppl 2), 44–50. http://dx.doi.org/10.1258/135581903322405153 Medline:14596747

Lomas, J. (1997). *Improving research dissemination and uptake in the health sector: Beyond the sound of one hand clapping.* Discussion document and recommendations prepared for the Advisory Committee on Health Services to the Federal/Provincial/Territorial Conference of Deputy Ministers, Canada, May 1997. Retrieved from http://www.cfhi-fcass.ca/migrated/pdf/mythbusters/handclapping_e.pdf

Martens, P. (2008). Building capacity in applied health and nursing services research in Canada: A seven year journey. *Healthcare Policy, 3*(special issue), 1–144.

Phaneuf, M.R., Lomas, J., McCutcheon, C., Wilson, D., & Church, J. (2007). Square pegs in round holes: The relative importance of traditional and non-traditional scholarship in Canadian universities. *Science Communication, 28*(4), 501–18. http://dx.doi.org/10.1177/1075547007302213

Acknowledgments

None of this would have been possible without the Canadian Health Services Research Foundation (CHSRF), now known as the Canadian Foundation for Healthcare Improvement (CFHI). As this book is retrospective, CFHI is referred to as CHSRF throughout. The chair awards were part of the Capacity for Applied Developmental Research and Evaluation in health services and nursing research (CADRE) program – a partnership between CFHI and the Canadian Institutes of Health Research (CIHR). Funding for the chairs was provided by CFHI, CIHR, and the following regional co-sponsors: Nova Scotia Heath Research Foundation, Ontario Ministry of Health and Long-Term Care, Ministère de la Santé et des Services sociaux du Québec/Fonds de recherche Santé du Québec, Winnipeg Regional Health Authority, and Alberta Innovates (formerly the Alberta Heritage Foundation for Medical Research).

Thanks also to Jyoti Phartiyal for technical expertise, without which the final manuscript would never have been completed.

SHAPING ACADEMIA FOR THE PUBLIC GOOD

Critical Reflections on the CHSRF/CIHR Chairs Program

PART ONE

Critical Reflections on the CHSRF/CIHR Chairs Program

Shaping Academia is about experimentation, innovation, and knowledge. The experimentation was the creation and implementation of a research, education, and mentorship chairs program developed by the Canadian Health Services Research Foundation (CHSRF), a federal government-funded research funding agency. A national competition was organized in the late 1990s and an international panel of experts adjudicated the selection of twelve chairs. During their ten-year tenures, they were to create innovative research programs with the explicit objectives to close the practice-research divide and educate and mentor the next generation of researchers to contribute to this enterprise. The innovation was in the creation of strong links between research, education, mentorship, and knowledge translation and exchange with health practitioners and decision-makers. Finally, knowledge was about the creation and, most importantly, passage from academia to the applied settings of health services and other decision-making organizations.

After the midterm review, the remaining eleven chairs began to talk about the valuable lessons we had learned through this experiment and the importance of sharing them. As a result, we decided to embark on a collective endeavour to reflect on our experiences. This book is the result.

Louise Potvin, the chair who took the lead in bringing us together around our exchanges through multiple drafts, wrote the introduction. As she explains, each chair selected our own focus, just as we did in applying for the program. But we shared our chapters with each other and debated their contents in ways that allowed us to create not a consensus but rather a collection that reflects both communal input and very different individual experiences. Beginning with the context that set the stage for the program, Potvin moves on to explore the five areas in which it was thought this experiment might have an impact.

In contrast, Chapter 2 exhibits the funder's perspective. Focusing on issues related to planning and implementing the chairs program, Erin (Morrison) Leith and Patricia Conrad describe how chairs tested a new approach to graduate training and research production. The expectations and outcomes were different for these chairs compared with traditional, research-based approaches. They explain how the "linkage and exchange approach" was the foundation on which chairs developed unique programs of research, training, and knowledge transfer. Researchers as knowledge producers used various engagement strategies to interact with decision- and policy-makers as research users. Leith and Conrad explore the challenges both chairs and CHSRF faced in adopting new and different ways to work together and the strategies they developed to address them. Finally, they reflect on the strategic and deliberate decisions taken by CHSRF and note what has worked well and what might be done differently, providing advice to others interested in replicating or adapting this approach.

1 Introduction: Reflections on an Innovation in Research Funding

LOUISE POTVIN

Shaping Academia is about innovation and knowledge. The innovation at the core of this book is the creation and implementation of a research, education, and mentorship chair funding program. This chairs program was developed at the end of the 1990s by the newly created Canadian Health Services Research Foundation (CHSRF) and was implemented in partnership with the Canadian Institutes of Health Research (CIHR). Twelve chairs were initially selected following a national competition. They were provided with funds and support to create research programs with the explicit goals of closing the gap between research, practice, programs, and policies in the health system, and of educating and mentoring the next generation of researchers to contribute to this initiative.

This innovation in research funding rested on the creation of strong links between an applied health services research platform, education and mentorship of graduate students and junior faculties, and knowledge translation and exchange with health organizations. Such goals were to be achieved by establishing lasting and extensive working collaborations between academic researchers, practitioners, and decision-makers in health organizations and government.

Finally, this book is about knowledge, its production in this innovative context, and its passage from academia to applied settings of health organizations. Once the midterm CHSRF/CIHR chairs program evaluation landmark was over, and about two-thirds of the way into its ten-year time frame, ten of the chairs decided to embark on a collective endeavour to reflect on the various aspects of their experience. *Shaping Academia* is the result of this collective reflection.

Defining the Innovation: Its Context, Objective, and Innovative Features

Research and its applications have become ever-present and extend human capacity in almost all areas of activity. Despite criticisms that research and technology generate risks that are inversely distributed as the wealth and progress they produce (Beck, 1992), science and scientific research are still generally associated with promises of improved living conditions and human progress, especially in health. Public demand for returns that are commensurate with expectations raised by science increases the pressure on researchers to develop knowledge with applications that contribute to solving the practical problems that arise in an increasingly complex society. To maintain and increase its level of funding, the research community has worked hard to shorten delays between the development of a hypothesis and its translation into technologies that improve aspects of life. The rise of the AIDS epidemic in the 1980s and the organization of the collective response to it, including that of the scientific community, provides an exemplar case of the social and political dynamics created when scientific knowledge and technology are called upon to solve novel and immediate threats (Dodier, 2003).

The Context: The Changing Landscape of Health Research Funding in Canada

The reorganization of health research funding in Canada at the end of the 1990s represents an effort to shift national research capacity towards a more problem-solving orientation. Until 1999, the Medical Research Council (MRC), together with two other national research funding councils, the Social Sciences and Humanities Research Council (SSHRC) and the National Science and Engineering Research Council (NSERC), were under the responsibility of the Ministry of Industry. The MRC was responsible for public funding of fundamental and clinical research, while Health Canada managed extramural research and development programs that essentially funded health services and population health research and demonstration projects. Since 2000, all medical and health research public money has been regrouped under CIHR, which has seen its budget tripled in comparison to that of the MRC. Contrary to the other councils, however, CIHR is now under the responsibility of the Ministry of Health, with a mandate to be more responsive to the needs of the ministry and other public policy-makers: "[CIHR] aims to excel according to internationally accepted standards of scientific excellence, in the creation of new health knowledge and its translation into improved health for Canadians, more effective health services and products, and a strengthened Canadian health care system" (Canadian Institutes of Health Research, 2011).

The significant rise in investments in research and scientific activity is coupled with increasingly pressing demands for immediate applications that improve population health, healthcare, and patients' quality of life. Scientific knowledge and research activity have to find applications outside of the laboratory, where they are produced at an increasingly fast pace. Researchers are no longer isolated in the role of knowledge producers whose work ends when their scientific publications are accepted. Instead, they are increasingly involved in the translation of knowledge into the improvement of human conditions.

The changes in health research funding opportunities in Canada were also coupled with a general increase in the number and variety of research funding programs. At the end of the 1990s, fostering Canada's leadership position in the knowledge economy was seen as a key investment for the budget surplus generated by the growing Canadian economy and federal administration reforms. Major investments were made throughout the whole spectrum of research needs and transformed the Canadian landscape. In terms of research personnel, the Canada Research Chairs program, launched in 2000, created 2,000 research chair positions in Canadian universities to support its research development strategic plan (Canada Research Chairs, 2011). To foster beginning research careers, the Millennium Scholarships Foundation, which operated from 1998 to 2008, distributed more than half a million bursaries to help students access post-secondary education (Campus Access, 2011). This program was replaced in 2009 by the Canadian Student Grant Program. To support the development of research infrastructure, foundations were also created, such as the Canadian Foundation for Innovation, which distributed close to $4 billion to support more than 5,500 projects in 128 Canadian research institutions during its first ten years of operation (Canadian Foundation for Innovation, 2008).

The impact that these new funding opportunities have had on the research capacity and organization of Canadian universities has yet to be studied. Observers of campus life, however, have witnessed spectacular growth in most universities in Canada in terms of undergraduate and graduate studentships, buildings, budgets, and faculty salaries as funding sources diversify with the increase of public and private investments. The role of the university as an institution has also changed during the past decades. Universities are increasingly called upon to help make sense of the ever-changing world that the knowledge they produce is creating. In a knowledge economy, universities are becoming key players, and those who steward the creation of knowledge – the researchers – are increasingly consulted and asked to contribute to the improvement of life and living conditions. The growth in the number of expert groups, think tanks, and expert task forces launched by governments, NGOs, and for-profit organizations, and in which researchers are asked to play a key role, is a sure sign that scientific and expert knowledge have acquired additional value in our globalized world. Given the imperatives to shorten delays between the production of scientific knowledge and its contribution to solving societal problems, research funding agencies are also trying to innovate and develop programs that will ensure a faster and greater uptake of scientific knowledge in the governance and management of public funds.

At the core of the innovation the CHSRF/CIHR chairs program represents is the notion of knowledge, its production, and its potential to improve the Canadian health system. Following its general uptake and success in the field of medical care, translating evidence-based practice into health system management and organization seemed like the logical thing to do. In addressing the problems faced by the Canadian health systems at the end of the past century, the National Forum on Health (1997) suggested that decision-makers and health practitioners needed to be equipped with the best evidence possible from empirical research and the mind set and conceptual tools needed to use it in their daily work. A corollary was that health research needed to be reformed to emphasize the applied problems practitioners and decision-makers face, and that future researchers needed to learn to work in close collaboration with those who would use their research. A complementary corollary was that the complexity of health systems and the problems they must address required multidisciplinary research. Such research is no longer confined to having nurses and physicians participating in the same project. Nowadays, multidisciplinary teams involve researchers from a wide range of scientific disciplines and from the social, life, and fundamental sciences.

The Objective: Closing the Knowledge-Practice Gap

In their work on knowledge production models, Gibbons and colleagues (1994) make a distinction between two modes of knowledge production. In Mode 1, knowledge is produced in laboratories and universities, apart from real world problems and in controlled situations, to discover universal truth. Scientific knowledge conceived in this way is in "epistemological rupture" with other kinds of knowledge and its superiority rests with its generalizability, reproducibility, and universality (Gibbons, 2000; Nowotny, Scott, & Gibbons, 2003). Roles are well defined for the main actors, who are either on the side of knowledge production, such as scientists and graduate students, or on that of knowledge use, such as practitioners and decision-makers. Scientists are meant to discover the laws that govern the world and express them in theories that form the hard core of scientific knowledge. Graduate students assist scientists and learn the ropes of their trade. Practitioners apply this knowledge after a period of professional training, composed mainly of lectures and practicum in which they have little contact with research. Decision-makers are supposed to use it as a rational substance to inform decision and policy.

In this orderly world, scientists, research apprentices, and scientific knowledge are not supposed to be influenced by practical problems. The narrow channel through which knowledge is transferred to practice is well guarded in university professional schools and regulated through professional accreditation bodies. This transfer is the paradigm of choice, and it is generally thought that knowledge remains unchanged throughout its passage from the world of science and research to that of practice and decision.

In sheer contrast, Mode 2 of knowledge production is characterized by five main attributes (Nowotny, Scott, & Gibbons, 2003). First, knowledge is generated within a context of application. Research is a problem-solving mechanism for questions that emerge from practice rather than from theoretical problems. Second, as it is driven by problems, research mobilizes all knowledge and methods relevant to the problem at hand in a transdisciplinary manner, meaning that there is no dominant disciplinary perspective. Third, a variety of actors produce knowledge in a diversity of heterogeneous sites. Fourth, research is reflexive. Conceived as being more akin to a conversation between research actors and research subjects than an objective investigation from a neutral knower, research leads to knowledge that is directly usable for acting on the researchable problem. Fifth, research is to be judged by novel quality control criteria that lie outside disciplinary boundaries and are of a more practical nature. Gibbons (1999) contrasts socially robust knowledge produced in Mode 2 with reliable knowledge produced in

Mode 1. The former is acceptable and useful outside of the scientific world, whereas the latter is only validated by disciplinary and expert internal criteria.

Although such a dichotomy between modes of knowledge production has the advantage of clearly differentiating research practices, the main criticism of this body of work is its lack of empirical foundation in sociological or anthropological studies of laboratories. More specifically, the contention that these two modes are incommensurable, that Mode 2 is replacing Mode 1 as an organization of scientific activity, and that the rupture between these two modes of knowledge production has not been substantiated by empirical observations (Shinn, 2002). Furthermore, according to Shinn (2002), usual descriptions of Mode 2 knowledge production seek to "minimize or to deny demarcations between academic, technical, industrial, political and social institutions. It thus dismisses boundaries and divisions of labour" (p. 604). This lack of differentiation between the constitutive elements of knowledge production systems makes it difficult to use those categories as foundations for a research program in the sociology of knowledge production.

The conception of knowledge production that underlines the innovative CHSRF/CIHR chairs program is akin to Mode 2 (Gibbons et al., 1994). Readers will find several references to this work throughout this book (see, for example, Chapter 12). However, the world of knowledge production, especially in the field of public health and health services research, has never been as orderly as Mode 1 implies, and the lack of differentiation associated with propositions about Mode 2 is a major impediment that will prevent capturing the whole of the chairs' collective experience with knowledge. As the chairs will show in this book, most of our programs were clearly identified as academic research operating in an applied world. We were clearly different and differentiated from our health system decision-making partners. In addition, the knowledge-practice gap that is at the core of the CHSRF/CIHR chairs program's innovations is not restricted to knowledge production; it also concerns sharing and diffusion. Throughout this book, we provide examples of how the wide range of activities developed within the chairs' programs, and for which knowledge was key, created bridges between research and practice and facilitated the circulation, use, and sharing of knowledge (Hartz, Denis, Moreira, & Matida, 2008).

The Innovation: The CADRE Program and the Chairs Program

CHSRF was created by the Canadian government in 1997 with an explicit mandate to contribute to the improvement and sustainability of the Canadian healthcare system by funding scientific research. Its mission was to support evidence-informed decision-making in the organization, management, and delivery of health services (Canadian Health Services Research Foundation, 2011a). As a new health research funding agency with an objective to help create strong links between the scientific community and the health system's decision- and policy-makers, and with limited resources, CHSRF had to create new funding mechanisms to fulfil its innovative mission. These mechanisms aimed to provide incentives for Canadian health services researchers to conduct research that was more directly relevant to policy- and decision-makers and practitioners.

One of CHSRF's first innovations was the Capacity for Applied and Developmental Research and Evaluation in Health Services and Nursing (CADRE), launched in 1999, which encompassed several innovative research funding practices. First, CADRE was a partnership between two newly created research funding agencies: CHSRF and CIHR. Apart from alliances with private enterprises, the idea of partnerships between several research funding agencies was rather new at that time in Canada. Second, CADRE has always been framed as the strategic response to the need to increase the Canadian capacity to conduct multidisciplinary research that would inform the health system's management and progress. Interestingly, CADRE aimed to change research practices with specific guidelines on how research should be conducted, leaving research themes and subjects somewhat open. It emphasized developing strong alliances and partnerships between academic researchers and health services decision-makers. It expected to increase the relevance of research and shorten the delay between knowledge production and its availability for decision-making. Third, CADRE was composed of four initiatives, each set to achieve specific objectives that would enhance capacity in applied health services and policy research (Canadian Health Services Research Foundation, 2011b).

As the first initiative to be launched, CADRE framed the chairs program as its flagship: "Chair Awards are an innovation in research funding. In addition to being mentors to students and junior faculty, the chairs are seen as resources for decision-makers at all levels who want to support an evidenced-informed approach in their areas of expertise" (Canadian Health Services Research Foundation, 2011c). Clearly, CADRE expected the chairs to develop an applied research platform that would produce usable and relevant knowledge for a health system's partner. This platform was to be used to mentor and educate graduate trainees and junior researchers, and to serve as a bridge for increased interactions and collaborations with the health system's decision-makers. (See Chapter 2 for a more complete description and analysis of CADRE and the chairs program.)

Following an open national competition, an international merit review panel composed of seasoned researchers and health system decision-makers selected twelve chairs. All chairs received a ten-year award, subject to a midterm review. All were launched between 2000 and 2001, and eleven were renewed following the 2005 and 2006 midterm review.

Three Areas of Impact for the Chairs Program

Having successfully implemented research programs that were to be vehicles for mentoring, education, and knowledge exchanges with health system partners, the chairs decided to collectively reflect on the experiences of the previous six or seven years. The ten chairs acted as ten loosely linked independent innovators, with big ideas about education, mentoring, and exchanges between academic researchers, health system practitioners, and decision-makers. Given CHSRF's strategic objectives with this program, there were commonalities and differences between each of the ten implementation sites. One of the chairs' first tasks was to adapt these big ideas to the unique circumstances in which they would implement them. Chair holders, their students, and their partners, as participants, had considerable freedom to develop and conduct research, mentoring, and knowledge exchange activities. More than seven years into this unique multi-site experiment, there was a need to analyse and examine how those chairs were individually and collectively creating new practices in research, graduate student mentoring, and knowledge exchange and translation with the intent to influence the decision-making process and professional practices within the health system.

Setting up mid-career academic researchers to work at the interface between academic knowledge production and health system decision-makers has led to numerous impacts at various levels. This book is an exploration of the innovations created by ten chairs in the process of implementing programs of research, mentorship, and knowledge exchange. Three fundamental questions guided our reflections on the lessons to be learned from our individual and collective experiences. One question pertains to the innovation in research practices: To what extent do research programs developed in close relationships with practice problems have to create new methods and ways to produce knowledge? Chairs have found various answers to this question. Some of us have found theoretical foundations in the literature on "engaged scholarship"; others have turned to Gibbons and Mode 2 research, or to "service learning." We did not attempt to find common threads across these various perspectives. Instead, we used this book as an opportunity to further explore some of the theoretical foundations of the research practices we implemented in response to the practical problems of our research program.

The second question relates to novel ways to structure learning and train researchers that match the demands for more multidisciplinary and flexible knowledge with the capacity to circulate much more rapidly in various arenas. Education was a major component of the CHSRF/CIHR chairs program and, contrary to other types of chair programs, CHSRF/CIHR chair holders needed to define strategic educational goals and devote significant parts of their budget to the pursuit of those goals.

The third question concerns the organizational and functional aspects of implementing innovations in academic and research environments. Chairs are academic structures for organizing research, education, and knowledge exchange, and so they require a certain level of organization to constrain and enable their work. Such organizational demands impact the conduct of academic careers, and we think that our atypical academic trajectories influenced our research environment, as well as that of our decision-maker partners.

Impact on Research and Research Practices

The first area of impact we focus on in this book is the practice of research. Increasingly research, especially applied research, is conceived as a practice that consists of the work of a community of actors to transform a reality. Collectively, and because of our commitment to developing research platforms that are relevant to health services' decision-making and practice, we, as chairs, have introduced many innovations in the practice of research.

In terms of governance, working closely with practice-based organizations and government has proven challenging, and we created many practical research governance tools. This challenge has impacted the organization of research as well as the governance of universities and science. Generally framed as an exclusive arena for researchers, other players who are struggling to integrate results are joining the research field. Several among us have created and used chair advisory boards with members beyond the usual academic suspects.

Also, in contrast to the loosely linked network of individuals that usually form a scientific community, the CHSRF/CIHR chairs program purposefully created multiple strong links between previously unrelated researchers in order to transform some of the research practices in the domains of health services and nursing research. The chairs developed areas of collaboration, some on substantive themes and research objectives, as is often the case in such projects. However, as a community of research practitioners facing similar process and implementation issues, we also developed new frames for analysing applied research practices. Despite the enormous variation among our programs, which ranged from health human resource management to cancer care to community health promotion, we were able to create connections among our practices.

Impact on Mentoring and Education Practices

The second area of impact we focus on in this book involves the mentoring practices of graduate and post-graduate students and junior faculty. Traditionally, the requirements of knowledge production bind and define the relationships between research mentors and their graduate students. Except for graduate program requirements, there is very little interference in the one-on-one mentoring relationship. One key parameter of the CHSRF/CIHR chairs program was the introduction of other non-scientist actors into this relationship. In the course of their graduate work, trainees in all chairs' programs had to learn to interact with a wide range of social actors with different relationships and attitudes towards scientific knowledge.

The chairs created a variety of arenas in which students could experiment with those relationships and develop their own research practices. Indeed, adding to the challenges of producing knowledge that was relevant to decision-makers, the chairs had to ensure that trainees would be able to satisfy the existing program requirements and the knowledge needs of decision-making partners.

Impact on Organizational Practices

The third area of impact is on organizations. The chairs program was a ten-year initiative, and so there was a sufficient built-in stability within the experiment to expect organizational impacts at three levels.

First of all, the chairs' innovative processes had an impact on universities as teaching and research institutions. In many instances the CHSRF/CIHR chairs program contributed to transforming academic life. One of the program's main thrusts was interdisciplinary research. More particularly, as a collective, the chairs built significant connections between health and social sciences. In current thinking, health and health systems are crossed by the same trends, values, and transformation forces that influence the societies in which they are produced and deployed (Kickbusch & McQueen, 2007). It is widely admitted that health cannot be reduced to a biological phenomenon and health systems are increasingly regarded as societal answers to bio-psycho-social problems. Understanding such complex objects requires interdisciplinary teamwork in which biomedical researchers work together with various types of social scientists.

In their current iteration, universities are generally ill equipped to promote and support interdisciplinary research endeavours or to train researchers to evolve in a complex environment. The departmental structure, in which academic careers are recruited, evaluated, and promoted according to criteria that stem from disciplinary work, is founded on disciplines of human knowledge. Any initiative that seeks to encompass researchers from various disciplines is bound to face not only cultural obstacles inherent to people whose languages and perspectives differ, but also structural and organizational barriers related to the way academic careers are conducted.

Second, the chairs program also had an impact on the health system itself. For the first time, in a concerted manner, a dozen research programs were launched with the deliberate objective to provide evidence to transform some of the health system's decision-making and professional practices, making them more responsive to, and integrated with, the results of scientific research. In addition, these research programs were selected based on their capacity to identify and involve relevant and powerful decision-makers in the planning and implementation of the research program. Each individual chair was an experiment in the conduct of applied research. The great variety of decision-making partners and health system organizations that were involved in the chairs speaks to the depth and width of the influence of the program in the Canadian health system.

Finally, the chairs program had a profound impact on academic careers. It was directed at mid-career academic researchers who had demonstrated interest and achievements in mentorship and knowledge transfer and exchange activities. We, as individuals, were given resources and recognition to create innovative structures within our institutions. We were engaged in an enterprise where the usual performance criteria applied to academic work expanded in the direction of applied training and knowledge transfer and exchange. If training was not necessarily a novelty in an academic career, knowledge transfer and the systematic establishment of close collaborations with decision-making and practitioner partners certainly were. We had to learn new ropes and develop new practices. Whole segments of our own training suddenly became irrelevant to the challenges we agreed to face. We navigated unknown waters and created new instruments to help us do so. For our colleagues who were aware of the trend towards closing the research-practice gap, we were precursors and innovators; for most of our colleagues, we remained strange animals whose frequent incursions outside of the university were often seen as a waste of time at best and a threat at worst.

The Reflexive Process of Creating This Book

Ultimately, *Shaping Academia* is about the practice of research and graduate education and how it can be transformed to better align with the needs of the health system. Intended as a critical reflection on the CHSRF/CIHR chairs program as implemented in different sites, this book represents the cumulative, collective learning of individuals who experimented with different ways to practice research and who developed and shared innovative tools as they did so. As an instrument in the pursuit of strategic objectives it had both pros and cons and we, as chair holders, are aware of and will report on both. We certainly do not want to advocate the CHSRF/CIHR chairs program as a model for research funding. However, there is no doubt that the program produced innovations in funding and research practices that have inspired others and helped to change the way research evidence and knowledge exchange are perceived.

Finally as a methodological consideration, readers should be reminded that the implementation sites varied greatly, and that there were some trends in the chair selection criteria. The ten chapters that form the core of this book make use of this variation to explore the various non-scientific networks in which knowledge circulates and is transformed.

This book is the result of our desire to collectively and critically analyse the process, implementation, and results of our chairs' programs in our attempt to contribute to the improvement of the health system. It is the result of a bottom-up process in which we each chose to reflect on a specific topic that emerged from our experiences. Over the course of two years, we met five times to design and refine a common frame to give meaning to our individual experiences, and to read and discuss each other's contributions. During those meetings, we candidly and openly reported our reflections on our own work. We held many discussions to clarify the parameters and critical dimensions of those experiments, as well as to develop common concepts and categories to help make sense of those case studies. This sharing process enriched each chair's understanding of our own programs and their impact. It did not, however, impose a common framework and a shared set of concepts for the analysis of each experience. Quite to the contrary, we each approached this project from our own disciplinary perspective using conceptual frameworks that allowed an in-depth analysis of the issues of concern.

Also noteworthy is the fact that CHSRF, as a funding agency, was an active participant in this reflexive project. Not only did it provide the funds necessary for the chairs to meet, but the CHSRF/CIHR chairs program officer took an active part in all of our discussions, providing at times a broader view of the experiment. The funding agency's involvement made this exercise akin to a participatory evaluation in which both experimenters and subjects confront perspectives in order to construct knowledge about the experience.

The book is composed of five parts. In Chapter 2, Erin (Morrison) Leith and Patricia Conrad present an extensive description of CHSRF's CADRE that provides a proper context for the chairs program. They also discuss how, throughout the program, CHSRF developed many innovative research management mechanisms that also shaped the implementation of the individual chairs.

As noted above, three general questions that correspond to the three main components of the chairs program (research, mentoring, and knowledge translation and exchange) guided our collective exploration of implementation challenges and areas of impact. Although most authors touch on all three areas, each focuses more directly on one specific area as a point of entry. The core of the book is thus composed of three parts. In Part 2, we focus on knowledge itself, its production, sharing, and its role in various applied settings. Very early in our reflection process, we realized that the knowledge we produced ended up in social arenas that we had not necessarily envisioned at the beginning of the program. Courts of justice, community organizations, and international NGOs represent relatively new actors in the circulatory systems of scientific health knowledge, and we were curious about the ways in which those actors interacted with, and transformed, this knowledge. In Part 2, we also reflect on the social organization of scientific knowledge and its role in modern society, and explore how constant dialogue between knowledge producers and users is redefining this role.

In Part 3, we discuss the novel ways to structure learning and education that various chair programs developed as a response to the demands of their various decision-making partners. The chairs provided infrastructure in which people at various stages in their academic careers could find training and mentorship and experiment with novel ways of interacting with knowledge and decision-makers, taking new risks or developing new networks.

In Part 4, we explore the practical organizational transformations that the chairs' programs spearheaded. One important focus is how our academic careers and lives were transformed participating in this experiment. After all, as Pat Armstrong writes in Chapter 10, we were not only chairs – we were also human beings with lives and careers of our own before CHSRF. In this collection of chapters, we reflect on how an academic trajectory that shifts to integrate knowledge users' perspectives can transform academic and health system practices. These transformations allow us to peek into the future of the academic life, in which the premise beneath the CHSRF/CIHR chairs program will prove true: collaboration and close work between research producers and users throughout the knowledge production and circulation process leads to more scientific input into decision-making and ultimately increases public program and policy's capacity to improve life and living conditions.

In Part 5, Lesley Degner, a chair whose agenda did not allow her to participate in the first series of meetings in which this book was created, concludes the volume. When she joined the last two meetings, Degner found great similarities between our discussions and her experiences. The distance she had from our analysis was such that she offered to use it to help us find some final collective lessons for the overall experiment.

A final word is required about the context of the CHSRF/CIHR chairs program. Although it was implemented in Canadian universities and institutions, the lessons learned and reflections made following this experiment can be of benefit beyond Canadian borders. First of all, although there are national variations in research funding programs and knowledge production organizational policies and programs, universities, as indicated in the word, are part of a project that transcends national borders. Scientific knowledge and its technological applications are intrinsic parts of the experience of modernity (Giddens, 1990), and we believe that this Canadian experiment could have been implemented with equal success in other Western societies. Second, a perusal of the reference lists at the end of each chapter will show that we borrowed extensively from scientific literature across North America, Europe, and Australia in order to analyse our experience. The innovations presented here should find echoes across Western societies in which research and research funding are part of national priorities.

REFERENCES

Beck, U. (1992). *Risk society: Towards a new modernity.* London: Sage.

Campus Access. (2011). *Canada Millennium Scholarships Program.* Retrieved September 2011 from http://www.campusaccess.com/financial-aid/scholarships-bursaries.html

Canada Research Chairs. (2011). *Program statistics.* Retrieved October 2011 from http://www.chairs-chaires.gc.ca/about_us-a_notre_sujet/statistics-statistiques-eng.aspx

Canadian Foundation for Innovation. (2008). *A decade of results through innovation.* Retrieved September 2011 from http://www.innovation.ca/10th

Canadian Health Services Research Foundation. (2011a). *Vision & mission.* Retrieved October 2011 from http://www.chsrf.ca/aboutus/visionandmission.aspx

Canadian Health Services Research Foundation. (2011b). *CADRE*. Retrieved October 2011 from http://www.cfhi-fcass.ca/whatwedo/applied researchandpolicyanalysis/cadre/cadrechairs.aspx

Canadian Health Services Research Foundation. (2011c). *CADRE Chairs*. Retrieved October 2011 from http://www.chsrf.ca/programs/cadre/cadrechairs.aspx

Canadian Institutes of Health Research. (2011). *Our mission*. Retrieved October 2011 from http://www.cihr.ca/e/7263.html

Dodier, N. (2003). *Leçons politiques de l'épidémie de SIDA*. Paris: Editions de l'École des hautes études en sciences sociales.

Gibbons, M. (1999). Science's new social contract with society. *Nature, 402*(6761 Suppl), C81–4. http://dx.doi.org/10.1038/35011576 Medline:10591229

Gibbons, M. (2000). Mode 2 society and the emergence of context-sensitive science. *Science & Public Policy, 27*(3), 159–63. http://dx.doi.org/10.3152/147154300781782011

Gibbons, M., Limoge, C., Nowotny, H., Schwartzmann, S., Scott, P., & Trow, M. (1994). *The new production of knowledge: The dynamics of science and research in contemporary societies*. London, UK: Sage.

Giddens, A. (1990). *The consequences of modernity*. Stanford, CA: Stanford University Press.

Hartz, Z.M.A., Denis, J.-L., Moreira, E., & Matida, A. (2008). From knowledge to action: Challenges and opportunities for increasing the use of evaluation in health promotion policies and practices. In L. Potvin, D.V. McQueen, M. Hall, L. De Salazar, L.M. Anderson, & Z.M.A. Hartz (Eds.), *Health promotion evaluation practices in the Americas: Values and research* (pp. 101–20). New York: Springer.

Kickbusch, I., & McQueen, D.V. (2007). *Health and modernity: The role of theory in health promotion*. New York: Springer.

National Forum on Health. (1997). Canada health action: Building on the legacy. (Vol. I). *The final report of the National Forum on Health*. Ottawa: National Forum on Health.

Nowotny, H., Scott, P., & Gibbons, M. (2003). "Mode 2" revisited: The new production of knowledge. *Minerva, 41*(3), 179–94. http://dx.doi.org/10.1023/A:1025505528250

Shinn, T. (2002). The triple helix and new production of knowledge: Prepackaged thinking on science and technology. *Social Studies of Science, 32*, 599–614.

2 Recipe for Innovation: Ingredients for an Applied Health Service Chair Model

ERIN (MORRISON) LEITH AND
PATRICIA CONRAD

It is said that old habits die hard. The same can be said of the steadfast traditions at the core of two previously exclusive worlds: academia and policy. A decade ago, Dr Jonathan Lomas and a few other self-professed renegades had a vision that they believed would shift traditions and result in systemic change in Canada's complex set of health systems. They considered several ingredients essential to achieve this ambitious vision. There would need to be:

- champions respected in both worlds prepared to drive the vision forward;
- researchers with established academic track records and a willingness to take risks;
- policy- and decision-making partners;
- a regional approach; and
- mentors to train the next generation of applied health services and nursing researchers.

This recipe for system change resulted in pan-Canadian innovation in capacity building for applied health services and nursing research, and for evidence-informed decision-making. In this chapter, from the perspective of the Canadian Health Services Research Foundation (CHSRF), we describe what worked well, what we forgot to add, and the modifications we suggest when recommending this recipe to others.

We begin this chapter with an overview of the historical occurrences that set the stage for the creation of CHSRF, including the partnership with the Canadian Institutes of Health Research (CIHR) and the establishment of the Capacity for Applied and Developmental Research and Evaluation (CADRE) program. We outline early assumptions and expectations of the program and its components, along with the underlying philosophies of linkage and exchange and merit review. We share lessons learned for those interested in embarking on similar capacity-building initiatives. We conclude with a discussion of what we anticipate will be garnered from a summative evaluation of the CADRE program and of the legacy of the CHSRF/CIHR Applied Health Services and Nursing Chairs.

Building Research Capacity: A New Era

Encouraged by the United Kingdom's research and development strategy of the 1990s, the Canadian government established an endowment to create a national foundation with a mandate to improve the scientific basis for decisions made by those who manage health system services (Secretary of State for Health, 1992). CHSRF was the realization of this vision. CHSRF was incorporated in 1997 with a mission to support evidence-informed decision-making in the organization, management, and delivery of health services. It developed various programs that predominantly focused on awarding funding to: (1) create new research knowledge through individual and team grants; (2) build research capacity through personal and institutional awards; and (3) transfer knowledge through CHSRF-led innovations in dissemination approaches that helped put research results directly into the hands of research users (Canadian Health Services Research Foundation, 2008a).

In 1999, the CHSRF Board of Trustees identified health system managers and policy-makers as the primary target audiences of the organization's work. The strategic focus on applied audiences has contributed to building CHSRF's international reputation as a leader for evidence-informed decision-making, knowledge transfer and exchange, and applied health services research (Hanney & González Block, 2006).

Merit Review Philosophy

A founding principle of equal representation for researchers and health system decision-makers has shaped the composition of CHSRF's board of trustees. One of CHSRF's first challenges as an organization was to design eligibility criteria and a review process to support the awarding of research grants and personnel awards to professional and academic individuals and teams across Canada.

CHSRF sought to advance the strategic alignment between research producers and end users and implemented the resulting merit review process in 1999. There are three key points in CHSRF's philosophy and approach to merit review. First, CHSRF's process gives equal weight to the research's potential impact on the health system and its scientific merit. Second, the long-term goal of CHSRF's research funding is not only to fund good quality health services research that has potentially high impact, but also to encourage and sustain ongoing links between health services researchers and relevant managers, decision-makers, and policy-makers. Third, the participation of, and input from, decision-makers in the planning and conduct of the research is an important consideration.

Fundamental innovations in CHSRF's overall funding philosophy include a requirement for applied health and nursing services researchers across Canada to partner with decision- and policy-makers, both to articulate the funding application and throughout the research process. With a merit review approach, CHSRF aims to shift health services research, which is historically investigator-driven, so that it is more applicable to health system policy-making. CHSRF assesses each research proposal through a merit review panel composed of an equal number of health services researchers, health system managers, and policy-makers. Since CHSRF adopted this approach, several other Canadian agencies have followed suit, including the Canadian Institutes of Health Research, the Canadian Patient Safety Institute, and the Nova Scotia Health Research Foundation.

CHSRF was considered well positioned to introduce merit review, which challenges how research funding was traditionally granted through well-known peer review processes. Initially, merit review encountered pushback from well-established Canadian health services researchers. Some referred to the new funding requirements as the "CHSRF hassle factor." Despite this early scepticism, many now embrace the merit review philosophy and cite the many advantages of actively working with decision- and policy-makers to conceptualize applied health services research. Health services researchers are enthusiastic when their research findings are incorporated into health system decision-making processes in an accurate and timely manner.

Call for Evidence-Informed Health System Decision-Making

In 1994, Canada's prime minister established the National Forum on Health to advise the federal government on innovative ways to improve

Canada's health system and the health of Canadians (Health Canada, 2004). The forum's final report (National Forum on Health, 1997) identified the inadequate use of research evidence in making decisions about the health system. It concluded that Canada needed to rapidly develop an evidence-based health system, with decisions made on the basis of appropriate, balanced, and high-quality evidence. By this time, the concept of evidence-based medicine was well established, and had a precipitating effect in identifying the need for the parallel practice of evidence-informed health system management in the Canadian context (Denis, Lomas, & Stipich, 2008). In support of this cultural shift, it was considered essential that researchers in applied health and nursing services learn to share their research findings and engage with health system policy- and decision-makers (Lomas, 2000).

While most academic graduate programs in Canada are built on a foundation of research methods, grant-writing skills, and traditional approaches of disseminating research findings (Smith & Edwards, 2003), they have largely ignored decision- and policy-makers as the end users of research. As graduate education programs are often discipline-based, the evolving multidisciplinary nature of applied health services research has gone unnoticed (Smith & Edwards, 2003). Another concern is that traditional pedagogical approaches continue to reinforce interactions with academic peers only. They are largely devoid of mechanisms that make it possible to interact with applied end users of research (Boyer, 1990; Lomas, 2000).

Although fostering skills for academic publishing is an essential element for productive and high-functioning applied health and nursing services researchers working in academic settings, Lomas (2000) and others have emphasized the various shortcomings of such training. Most notable is the incongruence between an emerging need to support research use in decision-making and the lack of student exposure to applied environments. This gap prevents students from understanding the limits of real-world access and application of research in health system decision-making (Lomas, 2000; Boyer, 1990).

Linkage and Exchange

As the inaugural chief executive officer of CHSRF, Jonathan Lomas began to write about tools and approaches he believed could bridge the gap between academia and health system decision-making. This became known as the CHSRF philosophy of linkage and exchange

Figure 2.1 CHSRF's Linkage and Exchange Philosophy

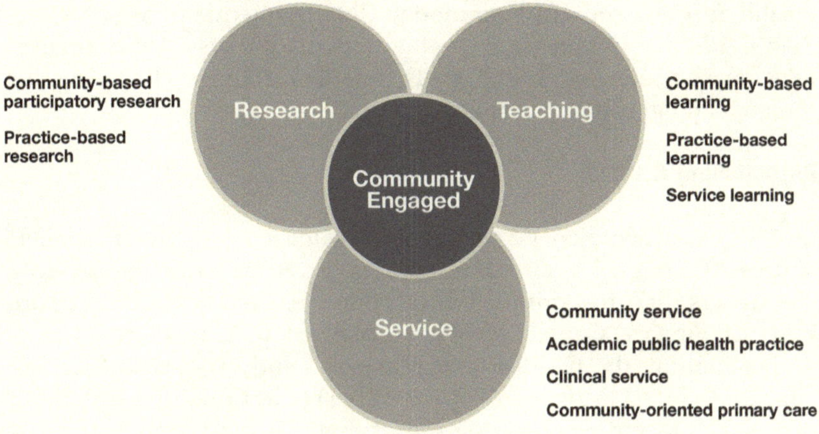

(see Figure 2.1). It stems from the underlying assumption that research evidence is an effective tool to improve health system decision-making. For this philosophy to become institutionalized in academic settings, there needed to be clear incentives for academic research and graduate training programs to recognize the value of up-front and ongoing engagement with decision-makers. CHSRF hypothesized that if the linkage and exchange philosophy was successfully integrated within academia, there would be a significant shift in recognition and reward practices for applied scholarship.

By 1999, linkage and exchange were ingrained in CHSRF's corporate culture. The board of trustees and merit review panels were comprised of health system decision- and policy-makers alongside respected health services and nursing applied researchers. It was assumed that engaging researchers with decision-makers on an ongoing basis, including during the selection process for research grants, would increase the use and applicability of research findings in health system and policy decisions. Ultimately, these encounters provide an opportunity for mutual understanding, and strengthen lasting relationships and trust between researchers and decision-makers (Lomas, 2000). The merit review panel, which unites decision-makers and researchers, is thought to be among CHSRF's most valuable capacity-building strategies.

Linkage and exchange is the key philosophical underpinning for the Capacity for Applied and Developmental Research and Evaluation in Health Services and Nursing model. CHSRF intended the pan-Canadian CADRE program to create the impetus for systemic change: to develop key knowledge and skills for linkage and exchange within research and graduate training programs.

Establishing CADRE

In 1999, the Canadian government awarded CHSRF $35 million to address the critical shortage of applied health and nursing services, researchers, and the production of policy-relevant research (Department of Finance Canada, 1999). Formalized in a memorandum of understanding, the CADRE program was jointly funded by CHSRF and CIHR over a thirteen-year period (1999 to 2012). At the end of this period, and including all partners' contributions, more than $80 million had been invested in applied health services and nursing research. CHSRF's contribution is subdivided into allocations from its core endowment fund and the Nursing Research Fund (NRF). The NRF, also announced in 1999, was a ten-year, $25-million investment from the federal government to allow CHSRF to build nursing research capacity in Canada (Department of Finance Canada, 1999). As steward of the NRF, CHSRF invested approximately $2.5 million per year for ten years (1999 to 2009), a portion of which supported the CADRE program in nursing research capacity development and research on nursing issues.

In 1999, the CADRE program represented an unprecedented ten-year funding agreement and had a mandate to "develop increased capacity in applied health and nursing services research in Canada" (Canadian Health Services Research Foundation, 2008b). CADRE's mandate was to produce more applied health and nursing services researchers, as well as to shift how training was delivered. It was designed to achieve these outcomes through interconnected funding components, including the Chair, Regional Training Centre (RTC), Postdoctoral (PDA), and Career Reorientation (CRA) Awards. The chairs program targeted mid-career academics with established research track records. CHSRF believed that senior-level personnel who had internationally recognized expertise, coupled with existing university infrastructure, could act as catalysts to accelerate the implementation and uptake of the linkage and exchange philosophy.

CHSRF was the designated administrative lead for CADRE and was responsible for program management and accountability. CHSRF has led evaluation efforts to date, including the midterm review of the CADRE program, which included an independent review of the Chair and RTC Awards. CHSRF staff also conducted a formative evaluation of the PDAs and CRAs between 2004 and 2006. CHSRF created numerous opportunities to actively engage the CADRE network, including through biannual meetings of the chairs and RTCs; ongoing support for transition and sustainability planning; oversight of the PDAs; and funding, planning, and hosting an annual event for health services and nursing research trainees.

CADRE Synergy

The CADRE program consisted of several interconnected components, or funding initiatives, that were designed to complement and address short- and long-term capacity needs on a regional basis. In 2000, CHSRF created three new competitions in which the newly awarded chairs were active as co-applicants, supervisors, and mentors. These competitions were:

- the first annual competition for the PDAs;
- the first annual competition for the CRAs; and
- a competition for RTCs designed to complement the distribution of capacity-building established through chairs.

Until the last competition, held in 2009, the annual PDAs offered recent doctoral graduates the training and experience necessary to launch an independent research career. Formal and informal interactions between the CHSRF/CIHR chairs and PDA candidates and recipients emerged almost immediately. Chairs served as primary and secondary academic supervisors and often helped postdoctoral applicants identify an appropriate decision-maker partner. Interactions between chairs and PDAs significantly expanded the chairs' network of applied researchers, drew talented researchers to the chair's academic institutions, and established lasting relationships with decision- and policy-makers attracted by the opportunity to generate new evidence.

The CRAs were aimed at individuals who wanted to shift the focus of their careers towards applied health or nursing services research. Again, numerous chairs acted as mentors to successful CRAs. However, because of declining interest, the CRAs were discontinued following a CHSRF Board of Trustees decision in 2007.

Finally, the RTC mandate is to increase accessibility to graduate-level education in applied health and nursing services research using a multi-university, interdisciplinary approach. The CHSRF/CIHR chairs have complemented the RTCs in various ways. Chairs were involved in the preparation of the RTC applications and continued to participate in curriculum development, program advisory committees, teach courses, run special institutes, and supervise RTC trainees' graduate research.

Much of the collaborative work that has emerged among the CADRE initiatives was anticipated, such as the natural tendency for chairs to mentor and supervise postdoctoral fellows and the collegiality between the chairs and RTCs. Other results were rather unexpected, such as the close ties of the chairs to the CHSRF Executive Training for Research Application (EXTRA) program, in which some of the chairs served as faculty and as academic advisors for health system improvement projects. The CADRE program has continued to evolve as each chair, RTC, and postdoctoral fellow adapts to the changing health services research landscape.

The CHSRF/CIHR Chairs Program

The CHSRF/CIHR chairs program was designed to "extend the scope of the traditional research chair or scientist model" (Canadian Health Services Research Foundation, 1999a) and build capacity for applied health and nursing services research in Canada. CHSRF intended to capitalize on the capacity and credibility of established researchers to fast track these efforts. This new senior award, with its ten-year duration, was the first of its kind and, as such, sought to foster a strong and long-term commitment between CHSRF, selected researchers, and those who would receive support, training, and mentoring throughout the program. The chairs were expected to encourage a linkage and exchange culture, increase use of evidence, and conduct policy-relevant research. The awards provided full salary and a program budget to support a program of research, education and mentoring, and linkage and exchange activities.

Decision- and policy-maker partners actively contributed to each chair's program of activities, a fundamental aspect of these awards. CHSRF believed such relationships were key to building locally sustainable capacity for evidence-informed decision-making within and across regions. Chair candidates were expected to attract cash and in-kind contributions from regional and national funding co-sponsors.

In keeping with the capacity-building mandate of CADRE, the chairs were required to allocate at least one-third of their time to mentoring trainees and junior researchers. In this way the linkage and exchange philosophy transferred from mentor to mentee. It was also reinforced with mandatory interactions between trainees and decision-makers, so that junior researchers gained an understanding of the needs of decision-makers and how they use research to promote evidence-informed decision-making.

The original objectives of the chairs program, as outlined in the 1999 Call for Letters of Intent (Canadian Health Services Research Foundation, 1999a), included:

- education and mentoring of the next generation of applied health and nursing services researchers (graduate and post-graduate students, junior faculty, and others seeking career renewal opportunities in the field), many of whom may be supported by future CHSRF-funded training awards;
- conduct research that holds promise to expand the quality and relevance of the evidence used in decision-making by policy-makers and health system managers; and
- linkage and exchange leadership to plan and implement dissemination and transfer activities that support the use of research by health system policy- and decision-makers.

The chairs program was intended to function across academia to bridge the gap between the world of research and that of decision-making. This ambitious mandate intentionally pushed the boundaries between academia and decision-makers' uneasiness about the use of research. CHSRF made several assumptions about these two worlds, and determined that research funders could shift the embedded traditions of both worlds to realize system-wide evidence-informed decision-making in Canada. During the design of the chairs program, a core set of obstacles were considered and strategies to overcome them implemented, including:

- Academic institutions neither traditionally nor sufficiently recognize and reward research partnerships. *The inclusion of community-based health system decision- and policy-makers as well as local co-funders in the chairs program was a concerted effort to promote the value added of a partnership model that involved multiple stakeholders.*

- Short-term research funding neither values nor provides the requisite time to establish and maintain decision- and policy-maker exchanges. *The ten-year funding horizon for the chairs program was designed to alleviate the pressure of constantly seeking out new funding and to guarantee stability.*
- Prior to the CHSRF Open Grants Competition and CADRE, granting agencies did not include incentives to foster linkage and exchange between research user/decision- and policy-makers and knowledge producers. *Dedicated resources were expected to help shift attention to how best to facilitate ongoing linkage and exchange.*
- Research literacy among decision- and policy-makers was low. *CHSRF envisioned the involvement of these community-based partners in the chairs program as an integral strategy aimed at enhancing participation skills by these partners over the lifetime of this award.*
- The majority of researchers lack the skills to communicate research results to decision- and policy-makers as well as to frame policy issues as research questions. *The chairs program provided funding and experiential training aimed at improving communication between the research and decision-making communities. They proposed that future researchers trained through the chairs program would receive mentoring on knowledge transfer strategies that promote the use of research evidence in health system decision- and policy-making.*
- Most research funding supported curiosity-driven research. *The ten-year funding timeline provided stability for chair holders and supported the involvement of health system decision- and policy-makers to establish joint research priorities.*
- There is a disconnect between researcher and decision-maker timelines for producing new knowledge. *The chairs program facilitated better alignment between the research and decision-making communities by encouraging decision- and policy-makers to think beyond the short term.*

Given the above, CHSRF worked to develop an award selection process that would address many of the issues stunting the growth of applied health and nursing services research in Canada.

The Chair Selection Process

CHSRF developed a review criteria and process to target experience, leadership, skills, and multiple types of partnerships for its unique awards. An international review panel of seasoned researchers, policy-makers, and senior research administrators provided rich perspectives on the qualities sought in the pool of candidates, added considerable lustre to the awards, and helped avoid a complex conflict of interest challenge. This panel experimented with non-traditional approaches to knowledge and research creation using the linkage and exchange model.

The competition was composed of two stages: initial letters of intent and invited full-scale applications (FSA). In the letters of intent stage, reviewers focused on scientific excellence, initial plans, and proposed partnerships. In the FSA stage, they focused on leadership, interpersonal and mentoring skills, and roles and commitments, both institutional and otherwise.

The FSA differed from the requirements to which traditional scientific research award competitions usually adhere. The CHSRF/CIHR chairs program diverted from tradition in several ways:

- CHSRF/CIHR enforced multi-level funding, and though it provided the majority of award funding, it also required support (either in-kind or monetary) from regional or provincial partners.
- Each chair's host institution was required to reinvest the equivalent of the chair's salary back into the program for the duration of the award.
- Chair applicants had to seek a funding agreement from the key stakeholders identified in the FSA. In addition to the host institutions, stakeholders included community partners such as health system decision- and policy-makers, and regional co-funders of applied health and nursing services research such as provincial research funding bodies. CHSRF considered this an important endorsement and commitment to the linkage and exchange philosophy.

The chairs program demanded an unprecedented level of involvement from community partners. In similar competitions, letters of support are commonly sought from community-based agencies or organizations that have a vested interest in the research outcomes. In the CHSRF/CIHR awards, the level of engagement transcended this standard letter of support. Instead, potential community partners worked with an applicant to decide how these relationships and collaborative efforts would unfold during the course of the proposed training and research program, and in what ways. For example, some community partners provided placements or internships for chair trainees, or forums and audiences in which trainees and chairs could translate and transfer research findings. In addition, the FSA required decision-maker partners to be drawn into the design of the chair's plan for knowledge production and research creation, and emphasized the need to rationalize proposed research projects. This unparalleled role brought a different dimension to the CHSRF/CIHR chairs by assuring that decision- and policy-making partners had a clearly defined stake in the proposed outcomes.

Although the involvement of regional funding co-sponsors was not novel, it did ensure the buy-in of local or provincial funding sources. However, the host academic institutions had an even more important role. The receipt of a traditional research chair award often provides academic institutions with additional resources and requires little or no support, other than usual infrastructure, in return. However, in a break with tradition, the merit review panel and consequently CHSRF/CIHR expected academic institutions to reinvest the freed-up salaries in the research program. The addition of this funding significantly increased the total budget available to the chairs and would subsequently be used to support related training and mentoring initiatives, including awards for graduate and postdoctoral fellowships, purchase of research associate time, and administrative support. This combination of CHSRF/CIHR support for the chair's salary and the host institution's reinvestment requirement tested the boundaries and established new rules between funders and university recipients. Over time, holding host academic institutions to account for their involvement in the CHSRF/CIHR chairs program proved to be an ongoing challenge for CHSRF and the chairs; each party had different expectations. As the chairs began to establish their programs, some host institutions struggled to deliver on the commitments outlined within the FSA, including infrastructure and communication support to publicize the awards and the work of the chairs, space, and human resources support to recruit administrative staff to manage these complex programs and partnerships.

To achieve more insight on candidates' suitability and leadership, CHSRF contracted a head-hunter firm to conduct over 200 interviews with references from five categories for each candidate invited to the second stage: a dean or vice president, a faculty colleague, another leader in the candidate's field, a current and former student, and a health system decision-maker. The firm summarized the conclusions from these interviews for each candidate, examining selected points and providing illustrative quotes from references. The results brought key perspectives into the process and influenced the final selection of candidates.

A list of the CHSRF/CIHR chairs is presented in Table 2.1. General characteristics of the chairs are as follows:

- Nine chairs began their awards in 2000, with four in nursing research and five in applied health services research.
- Three chairs began their awards in 2001, with one in nursing research and two in applied health services research.
- The chairs were 75 per cent female and 25 per cent male.
- Geographically, there was one chair in Nova Scotia, three in Quebec, six in Ontario, one in Manitoba, and one in Alberta.
- There were four chairs from nursing, and one chair each from health economics, sociology and women's studies, and mental health.
- Chairs were selected from a wide range of health services and social sciences backgrounds, including pharmacy, public health, political science, and organizational behaviour.

As of 2008, CADRE had produced more than 1,249 applied health services and nursing researchers. Of this number, the chairs cumulatively sponsored and mentored 723 trainees. The chairs' trainees vary considerably by discipline, but can generally be categorized into three distinct groups: social sciences (13 per cent, 92), nursing (46 per cent, 333), and health sciences (34 per cent, 250). CADRE trainees range from novice researchers to established mentees, but most commonly include junior faculty (5 per cent, 28), and are postdoctoral fellows (9 per cent, 51), master's candidates (21 per cent, 116), or doctoral candidates (38 per cent, 205). These figures for health services, policy, and nursing trainees reflect similar gender stratification to that of the chairs, which was 86 per cent female and 13 per cent male.

Framing the CHSRF/CIHR Chairs Program as a Natural Experiment

Granting agencies can promote cultural shifts. During the late 1990s, CHSRF and CIHR were convinced that the linkage and exchange philosophy was a promising way to address deficiencies in the use of applied health and nursing services research to support evidence-informed decision-making (Lomas, 2000). In 1999, to advance understanding of the philosophy, CHSRF convened a national workshop in which Canadian researchers and decision-makers, along with national

Table 2.1 Description of CHSRF/CIHR Chair Holders

Full Name	Host Unit	Administering Institution	Province	Chair Title	Discipline	Chair Start and End Date*	Decision-Maker Partners
Pat Armstrong	Department of Sociology and Women's Studies, Faculty of Arts	York University	Ontario	Women and Health Services: Policies and Politics	Sociology	2001–2011	• Women's Health Bureau, Health Canada • Canadian Federation of Nurses Union
Peter C. Coyte	Department of Health Policy, Management, and Evaluation, Faculty of Medicine	University of Toronto	Ontario	Health Care Settings and Canadians: A Program of Research, Education, and Linkage	Health Economics	2000–2010	• Homecare Evaluation and Research Centre • Comcare Health Services • St Elizabeth Health Care • VON Canada • We Care Home Health Services • Canadian Healthcare Association • Canadian Homecare Association • Canadian Association for Community Care • The Change Foundation • Heart and Stroke Foundation of Ontario

Lesley Degner	Faculty of Nursing	University of Manitoba		Development of Evidence-Based Nursing Practice in Cancer Care, Palliative Care, and Cancer Prevention	Nursing	2000–2010	• Centre for Behavioural Research and Program Evaluation, University of Waterloo
Jean-Louis Denis	Health Administration Department, Faculty of Medicine	University of Montreal	Quebec	Governance and Transformation of Health Care Organizations	Organisational Behaviour	2000–2010	• Régie régionale de la santé et des services sociaux de Montreal
Alba DiCenso	School of Nursing, Department of Clinical Epidemiology and Biostatistics, Faculty of Health Sciences	McMaster University	Ontario	Evaluation of Advanced Practice Nursing Roles and Interventions	Nursing	2001–2011	• Ontario Ministry of Health and Long-Term Care (Nursing Secretariat)
Nancy Edwards	School of Nursing, Faculty of Health Sciences	University of Ottawa	Ontario	Multiple Interventions in Community Health Nursing Care	Nursing	2000–2012	• Ottawa-Carleton Health Department • Sisters of Charity of Ottawa Health Service
Paula Goering	Health Systems Research and Consulting Unit	Centre for Addiction and Mental Health	Ontario	Generating and Disseminating Best Practices in Mental Health and Addictions	Nursing/ Mental Health	2000–2010	• Ontario Ministry of Health and Long Term Care (Mental Health and Rehabilitation Reform Branch)

(continued)

Table 2.1 continued

Full Name	Host Unit	Administering Institution	Province	Chair Title	Discipline	Chair Start and End Date*	Decision-Maker Partners
Réjean Landry	Management Department, Faculty of Administrative Sciences	Laval University	Quebec	Knowledge Transfer and Innovation	Political Science	2000–2010	• Ministère de la santé et des services sociaux du Québec
Linda O'Brien-Pallas	Nursing Health Services Research Unit, Faculty of Nursing	University of Toronto	Ontario	Nursing Human Resources for the New Millennium	Nursing	2000–2010	• Ontario Ministry of Health and Long-Term Care
Louise Potvin	Department of Social and Preventive Medicine, Faculty of Medicine	University of Montreal	Quebec	Community Approaches and Health Inequalities	Public Health	2001–2011	• Montreal Public Health Directorate
Ingrid Sketris	College of Pharmacy, Faculty of Health Professions	Dalhousie University	Nova Scotia	Developing and Applying Drug Use Management Strategies and Policies for Nova Scotia's Provincial Drug Programs: A Partnership of Researchers, Health Care Professionals, Consumers, and Government	Pharmacy	2000–2011	• Nova Scotia Department of Health

and provincial research funders, considered implementation issues (Canadian Health Services Research Foundation, 1999b). Participants identified key differences between how the research and decision-making communities might use linkage and exchange to connect. They also identified unique features of both environments, which informed the funding, award structure, and program requirements that underpin the chairs program.

Furthermore, the group of awarded chairs and their programs, research models, partners, and institutions were considerably diverse (see Table 2.1). As the chairs program was a pilot program, CHSRF planned to learn and share the chair experience with funders and individuals interested in this form of capacity development. Consequently, CHSRF funded semi-annual meetings in which the chairs could problem solve and share progress, challenges, and new ideas. Early meetings focused on:

- building familiarity between the chairs;
- understanding immediate challenges and identifying where and how CHSRF could help (e.g., institutions that did not honour infrastructure commitments, grants offices that challenged linkage and exchange expenditures, chairs unable to divest themselves of other responsibilities);
- introducing topics identified by reviewers (e.g., strategic advisory committees, accountability); and
- identifying potential collective work (e.g., mentorship and early thoughts on program evaluation models).

The CHSRF/CIHR Chairs Program versus the Traditional Scientist Model

The chairs program was intended to push the boundaries of a traditional research chair or scientist model. The CHSRF/CIHR chairs program differed from many traditional scientist awards in that award holders dedicated a significant proportion of their program – approximately two-thirds – to education, mentoring, and knowledge transfer. These expectations depart from usual academic outputs in that they promote real-world engagement with community-based health and policy decision-makers through linkage and exchange.

The CHSRF/CIHR chairs program recognized that outstanding research expertise and credible peer-review papers and research grants enabled the chairs to pilot this new approach. However, the anticipated outcomes for the program extended far beyond traditional academic outputs such as publications in peer-reviewed journals and papers at peer-reviewed conferences. The CHSRF/CIHR chair model seeks to ensure research is applied, and so effectively promotes balance between health system decision- and policy-making and the natural career interests of university-based researchers.

The CHSRF/CIHR chairs program activities differ substantially from those of traditional research activities, a fact that has become more apparent since its inception. Most notable at the outset was the equal priority given to education and mentoring, knowledge transfer, and producing new knowledge through research. More traditional research awards focus on producing research for consumption by predominantly academic audiences, where it is taken for granted that selected trainees will receive mentoring as part of the process. In contrast, CHSRF/CIHR chairs were expected to devote significantly less time to the role of lead investigator and more time to ensuring their trainees acquired relevant, quality research experience throughout all research phases, from identification of research goals and design to proposal writing to execution to publication and beyond.

Chair holders were required to continuously look to their partners for opportunities to share knowledge in non-traditional ways (for example, through newsletters, web postings, face-to-face meetings, and fact sheets). These approaches seem to mirror decision-makers' preferences concerning access to research results. The awards targeted tenured applied health and nursing research professors with established track records in research. This was deliberate, as university-based tenure and promotion committees continue to place a higher value on traditional methods of dissemination that centre on peer review, despite the fact that the linkage and exchange model has become accepted as a viable approach.

CHSRF/CIHR chairs were also required to conduct strategic and concerted recruitment of diverse, interdisciplinary program participants. Moreover, chairs were expected to mentor and educate their trainees by directly involving them in their research, as well as by creating new program delivery infrastructures to attract new trainees through relevant educational programs, courses, internships, and so on. Many chairs actively engaged with, and to some extent relied on, their community-based partners for these opportunities and strategies. As a result, the chairs invested significant time in new program development, which is a departure from the more traditional science model in which the strength of existing infrastructure is often a critical factor in becoming a successful research applicant.

Unlike in the traditional science model, CHSRF deliberately linked chairs to each other by providing ongoing funding for a chair's network that met twice yearly. In addition, CHSRF viewed chairs as an important source of regional intelligence and expertise and involved them in its activities and initiatives, such as the popular CHSRF Mythbusters article series, the "Listening for Direction" consultations, annual workshops, and the EXTRA program, as well as seeking their advice based on their research expertise. This ongoing engagement between CHSRF as a funder and its chairs has formed greater connections with other national initiatives. These add-on expectations depart from the traditional scientist chair model, where submitting an annual progress report is often the only involvement the grant funder has with a recipient.

In terms of reporting, the CADRE program, and the chairs program within it, was introduced at a time when accountability had become an increasingly important and politically sensitive issue for funding agencies and their partners. Chairs who were accustomed to limited reporting found CHSRF's hands-on approach overbearing. CHSRF required chairs to prepare an annual progress report on their objectives, an accountability framework report, an update on demographic and trainee data, and financial statements from the host institution. Chairs also prepared significant documentation to inform the CADRE midterm review and later transition plans. This is in addition to the reporting chairs submitted to their advisory committees and institutions. CHSRF and the chairs struggled to find the right balance between quantitative and qualitative reporting to fulfil accountability needs and ensure timely and efficient sharing of information.

Reporting structures also highlighted another area of learning: the optimal balance of time and energy between research, training and mentoring, and linkage and exchange work with health system partners. The initial vision of this program failed to appreciate the high degree of positive exchange between these focuses and the critical nature of the research platform for training and mentoring. It also took time for many of the chairs to appreciate how a research manager or executive secretary might help them juggle the growing facets of research, training, and health system and funding partnerships.

Adoption of the CHSRF/CIHR Chairs Program Model

The chairs program began during a period of transition in the health research landscape. Since CADRE was first conceptualized, the number and nature of health services research funders has dramatically increased. Prior to 2000, only a handful of national and provincial health services research funders existed in Canada.

Amidst the complex landscape of funders, CHSRF was in a unique position to influence similar organizations as they began to develop health services funding strategies. Linkage and exchange, no matter what you call it – knowledge transfer, translation, use, or mobilization – is now integrated into the funding mechanisms for applied health services research in Canada. For example, since entering the funding landscape in 2000, CIHR's overall mandate has shifted to emphasize knowledge translation. This integration is particularly evident within the Institute of Health Services and Policy Research (IHSPR), which works closely with CHSRF and requires grant recipients to establish linkages between health researchers and application settings.

The CADRE program model has influenced other programs: the Aboriginal Capacity and Developmental Research Environments (ACADRE) program at CIHR's Institute of Aboriginal Health is directly modelled on CADRE (Canadian Institutes of Health Research, 2007), and in 2008, CIHR's Institute of Population and Public Health (IPPH) and IHSPR both granted new chair awards expressly modelled after the CHSRF/CIHR chairs program. IHSPR awarded seven junior chairs (Canadian Institutes of Health Research, 2008a) and IPPH targeted mid-career faculty, funding fifteen applied public health chairs (Canadian Institutes of Health Research, 2008b). Similar to the CHSRF/CIHR chairs, these new chairs conduct policy-relevant research, share it with decision-makers, and educate and mentor the current and next generation of public and health services researchers (trainees, postgraduate students, and junior faculty), practitioners, and policy-makers. These new chairs have the benefit of better understanding the advantages and disadvantages, as well as the challenges, that accompany a linkage and exchange philosophy in an academic, and even decision-making, world that is not structured to support it. The CHSRF/CIHR chairs have also engaged with these new chairs, and are looking for ways to share their experience with this new generation.

Various national, provincial, and international organizations have adopted and continue to adapt these innovative approaches to integrate evidence-informed decision-making into health systems. For example, the Canada Research Chairs program began shortly after CADRE and brought a major influx of chair-based funds – $900 million to support more than 2,000 chairs – with a central focus on research excellence into a large number of institutions. The CHSRF/CIHR chairs were clearly overshadowed by this initiative, and their host institutions may have been more attentive to the larger program, which brings them more research personnel.

This is the realization of a long-term outcome of the CADRE program: that both funders and academic institutions would adopt the linkage and exchange philosophy. The next feat will be to successfully integrate linkage and exchange activities into the reward and recognition structure of the university promotion and tenure process.

Reflections from a Funder's Perspective

CHSRF has been fortunate and, in many ways, successful in building capacity for applied health services and nursing research in Canada while advancing the integration of the linkage and exchange philosophy within academic institutions. Much of this credit lies with those who have borne the brunt of the work – the award recipients. From master's students to postdoctoral awardees, and from junior faculty mentees to senior career scientists, those that comprise the CADRE network have, by virtue of the applied nature of their research, narrowed the gap between academia and policy.

As a new organization, CHSRF was lucky to have a passionate and committed CEO in Jonathan Lomas, a leader to whom researchers and decision-makers alike could relate. With the leadership and vision for the CADRE program secure, there was considerable latitude in how each component could develop operations. CHSRF was, after all, a new organization claiming to be an innovative incubator. As an organization, it has learned many lessons throughout the last decade as the planning, coordinating, and administrative lead for the CADRE program.

The following are reflections from a funder's perspective about key lessons CHSRF has garnered from this experience. They provide insights about what has worked well and why, where we might have benefited from hindsight, and our advice to others.

What Worked

Stability in funding. The chairs frequently cite the tremendous benefit of having a ten-year funding period. A decade of stable funding allowed them to develop exceptional training and mentoring programs, as well as renowned research programs and lasting relationships with health system decision- and policy-makers, resulting in more evidence-informed decision-making.

International merit review. The international merit review panel approach used during the chairs program selection process added prestige and increased the profile of recipients. Some refer to this as the name-on-the-door effect, which presented opportunities for the CHSRF/CIHR chairs to gain access to a pan-Canadian network of health services and nursing research experts and grab the attention of health system decision- and policy-makers.

Network development. From the inception of the program, both CHSRF and CIHR provided administrative support funding for biannual network meetings for the chairs and RTCs. While the chairs established their research and mentoring programs, these meetings allowed them to interact, share experiences, and formalize the group as a pan-Canadian network. As the program matured, these meetings begun to expand the collaboration between the chairs, including on collective legacy pieces such as this book.

Hands-on funders. The exchange between funders and the chairs was of further benefit. The chairs' involvement in additional linkage and exchange activities led by CHSRF helped them become acculturated to this model of collaborative research production; the chairs and their trainees have been very successful in many CIHR national funding competitions.

Partnership between co-funders. The memorandum of understanding between CHSRF and CIHR set out important processes for the CADRE program. It continues to be an important historical document used by CHSRF to reinforce roles and responsibilities of the funders and various program requirements, including review and evaluation points. Assigning administrative leadership to CHSRF provided clarity of communication and one single contact point.

Monitoring performance. The annual reporting requirements involved submitting to CHSRF: (1) an updated participant database; (2) financial statements and expenditure forecasts; and (3) a program report that described progress and annual achievements. This documentation continues to provide baseline information about the evolution of each chair and presents chronological data for the reviewers to judge progress against program objectives.

Lessons Learned

Not everything went exactly as planned. Over the course of a decade, the nature of the CADRE program made it impossible to predict every issue related to the number of partners, regional factors, and organization.

Tracking participant data. A participant database tracking trainee involvement and outcomes was developed soon after CADRE was launched. The chairs were required, in compliance with their award conditions, to submit information annually about their trainees. Due to a lack of consistent definitions and data collection methods, difficulties in tracking student achievements were identified during the midterm evaluations. This central database was then modified and was actively managed by CHSRF to ensure student outcomes were accurately reported.

Canadian training environment. CHSRF did not undertake an environmental scan of existing applied health and nursing services graduate programs prior to developing CADRE. This baseline information could have been a valuable way to document retrospectively how the program and related graduate training opportunities affected various training gaps.

Promotion and branding. As the coordinating and administrative lead for CADRE, CHSRF could have taken a more active approach to promoting and branding the program and its components. The co-leads of the CADRE midterm review noted this need. Since 2006, CHSRF has established a CADRE brand, created an official electronic newsletter of the CADRE network, and promoted the work of the chairs, RTCs, and PDAs to Canadian and international audiences.

Sustainability and transition planning. It seems counterintuitive to think about how a program might sustain itself prior to becoming fully operational. Introducing the notion of legacies and planning in relation to program continuity, where feasible, could have prompted more timely consideration of how the chairs might have promoted themselves to spread awareness of this chair model. However, despite limited interest from the chairs themselves, CHSRF encouraged them to self-promote by developing strategic advisory committees and sorting strategic priorities.

Early evaluation. Although the original CADRE planning documents indicated major evaluation milestones, a comprehensive evaluation plan was not articulated until the last several years of the program. At times, the lack of evaluative evidence has resulted in a lack of data to support the development of new program directions that could have benefited from a clear understanding of CADRE's accumulating impact.

Conclusion and Advice to Others

CHSRF's experience in creating, implementing, and evolving with CADRE and the chairs was truly an innovation that has advanced the notion of applied research and research use in academia and policy. Since 1999, CHSRF has learned many lessons and is a wiser organization for its collaboration and partnership through the CADRE program. The recipe for linkage and exchange seemed to resonate with some, and although it sometimes faced resistance, few, once exposed, have returned to traditional investigator-driven research. Rather, academics and decision-makers alike cite the many advantages and opportunities presented to them through a collaborative approach, which they feel is worth the extra time and effort.

CHSRF offers the following advice for those developing a similar program to contemplate:

- the need to balance the funder's role as a granting agency and its role in a partnership in which both parties are open to learning and adapting along the way;
- the need for consistency of data requirements and comparable features across programs and the need for flexibility and creativity in program design and development;
- the need for the funder and recipients to respect aspects of formal accountability and also efforts to innovate. Although flexibility and innovation can be both strengths and weaknesses in any program, there needs to be tolerance and leadership in the right quantities and qualities on both sides of this equation;
- the significance of situating a chair program within a strong research milieu where there is a high value placed on knowledge transfer and research use;
- the need to enhance trust and collaborative horizontal and vertical relationships through face-to-face network development and site visits;

- the need to clearly specify and promote performance monitoring and accountability to provoke strategic thinking and expectations; and
- the importance of networking support.

Investing in capacity building requires strong and wise leadership and skills that bridge the gap between the academic world and health systems. We hope the description of this natural experiment and our experience as funders is of value to others contemplating a similar approach.

Acknowledgments

Special thanks to Linda Murphy, who made a significant contribution to this chapter in writing and in legacy as the inaugural CADRE program lead.

REFERENCES

Boyer, E. (1990). *Scholarship reconsidered.* New York: The Carnegie Foundation for the Advancement of Teaching.

Canadian Health Services Research Foundation. (1999a). *Initial call for letters of intent for CHSRF/CIHR chairs.*

Canadian Health Services Research Foundation. (1999b). *Issues in linkage and exchange between researchers and decision makers.*

Canadian Health Services Research Foundation. (2008a). *Statement of institutional purpose.* Retrieved 17 March 2008 from http://www.chsrf.ca/about/do_statement_purpose_e.php

Canadian Health Services Research Foundation. (2008b). *Capacity for Applied and Development Research and Evaluation (CADRE).* Retrieved 17 March 2008 from http://www.cfhi-fcass.ca/whatwedo/appliedresearchandpolicyanalysis/cadre.aspx

Canadian Institutes of Health Research. (2007). *Aboriginal Capacity and Development Research Environment (ACADRE).* Retrieved 2009 from http://www.cihr-irsc.gc.ca/e/4103.html

Canadian Institutes of Health Research. (2008a). *Applied chairs in health services and policy research.* Retrieved 2009 from http://www.cihr-irsc.gc.ca/e/37826.html

Canadian Institutes of Health Research. (2008b). *Applied public health chair.* Retrieved 2008 from http://www.cihr-irsc.gc.ca/e/35106.html

Denis, J.L., Lomas, J., & Stipich, N. (2008). Creating receptor capacity for research in the health system: The Executive Training for Research Application (EXTRA) program in Canada. *Journal of Health Services and Policy, 13*(Suppl 1), 1–7. http://dx.doi.org/10.1258/jhsrp.2007.007123 Medline:18325161

Department of Finance Canada. (1999). *Budget 1999, strengthening health care for Canadians.* Ottawa: Department of Finance Canada.

Hanney, S.R., & González Block, M.A. (2006). Building health research systems to achieve better health. *Health Research Policy and Systems, 4*(1), 10–16. http://dx.doi.org/10.1186/1478-4505-4-10 Medline:17087830

Health Canada. (2004). *National forum on Health Canada's health infrastructure.* Retrieved October 2011 from http://www.hc-sc.gc.ca/hcs-sss/ehealth-esante/infostructure/nfoh_nfss-eng.php

Lomas, J. (2000). Using "linkage and exchange" to move research into policy at a Canadian foundation. *Health Affairs (Project Hope), 19*(3), 236–40. http://dx.doi.org/10.1377/hlthaff.19.3.236 Medline:10812803

National Forum on Health. (1997). *Canada health action: Building on the legacy* (Vol. 1). Ottawa: Health Canada.

Secretary of State for Health. (1992). *Health of the nation: A strategy for health in England.* London: Her Majesty's Stationery Office.

Smith, D., & Edwards, N. (2003). Innovation: Building research capacity. *The Canadian Nurse, 99*(9), 23–7. Medline:14621530

PART TWO

Innovations in Research Practices

With large public investments especially in health research, there were increasing demands for new strategies to link promising scientific results to the development or improvement of goods, services, practices, and policies. CHSRF, and the chairs program, was in large measure dedicated to promoting more systematic linkages and exchanges between researchers and decision-makers, a process labelled knowledge transfer.

Knowledge transfer as a field of practice and research has evolved dramatically over the last twenty years. In Chapter 3 in this section, Réjean Landry and collaborator Nabil Amara illustrate how the dialogue between policy-makers and researchers has been instrumental in the evolution of the understanding of and conceptual approaches to knowledge transfer. To begin, they present the traditional knowledge transfer models and their associated policy models before discussing knowledge transfer through commercialization and knowledge spillovers. Next, they examine the complementary relationship between the production of research knowledge and its transfer outside the academic community. Finally, they raise the issue of knowledge management and argue that policy interventions focused on individuals are not sufficient to lead to the expected levels of transfer. In addition, knowledge transfer requires a focus on organizations and how knowledge is managed through various organizational processes. In the conclusion, they address a question raised by an increasing number of managers: "How can a large organization create or increase value from the use of knowledge?"

In Chapter 4, Peter C. Coyte discusses the activities of the chairs program in the cultivation and advancement of evidence for policy decision-making. He focuses on just one aspect of the role of evidence in influencing policy and practice; specifically, that within law and Canadian jurisprudence. He discusses two exemplars: first, the pedagogic role for evidence creation and knowledge dissemination within the chairs program, and second, the evidence concerning immigration policy. The first exemplar highlights research as a platform for education and mentoring activities as well as for knowledge translation, while the second highlights tensions associated with a shift from curiosity-driven research to a more directed series of activities. He stresses non-traditional mechanisms for knowledge translation and describes the enhanced learning experience for trainees who are active participants in the creation and dissemination of knowledge. He concludes with a range of important knowledge translation lessons.

In Chapter 5, Louise Potvin argues that research can play a crucial role in supporting the transformation of the often-conflicted relationships between government agencies and community organizations. In addition to being on two opposite sides of the funding equation, government agencies and community organizations operate in very different modes. Their interactions take place in a highly politicized space, and when research becomes a third key actor in that space, it incorporates two major elements. The first is distance from the action, which is necessary for the development of a reflexive perspective that allows actors to reconsider various actions from a different point of view. The second is knowledge as a resource and an orientation for action. The focus on the inclusion of knowledge facilitates the passage from a space for prescription to an experimental arena leading to innovation. Social health is thus a space of conflicting cooperation between state agencies and community organizations in which the inclusion of a research partner facilitates reflexivity and innovation. Potvin examines some of the conditions that enhance the capacity for research to play such a role in the socio-health space.

In the final chapter in this section, Linda O'Brien-Pallas and collaborator Lauren Hayes explore the conceptual inadequacy of the models for estimating human resource requirements for nursing. They reveal the chairs program's emphasis on working with governments and other decision-makers for research-based change. They argue that the use of simple supply models has contributed to numerous swings between shortages and surpluses of nurses. Even though policy-makers have identified health human resources (HHR) as a major priority area for health services research, approaches to nursing have traditionally been plagued with methodological and conceptual limitations. Based on this chair's experiences in advancing the underdeveloped science of HHR planning, and drawing on relevant literature, they describe the journey from developing an HHR conceptual framework to using study findings in HHR planning and policy. They highlight some completed studies that have influenced HHR policy in nursing and set out the health human resource framework. They then consider the role of linkage and exchange and the challenges of bringing together researchers and decision-makers in the research process and in application.

3 From Knowledge Transfer to Knowledge Management and Value Creation

RÉJEAN LANDRY IN COLLABORATION WITH NABIL AMARA

In the first section of this chapter, we review how the research, networking, and training program of the CHSRF/CIHR Chair in Knowledge Transfer and Innovation emerged and progressively evolved over time. In the second section, we examine some of the major changes in the way researchers, notably researchers associated with the chair in response to policy-makers' expectations and concerns, conceptualized knowledge transfer. In the third section, dealing with knowledge management, we stress the fact that policy interventions that focus on individuals are insufficient to create the expected levels of transfer, and that one has also to pay attention to organizations and how knowledge is managed through various organizational processes. In conclusion, we address a recent question raised by an increasing number of managers: "How can a large organization create or increase value from the use of knowledge?"

A Brief History of the Chair's Accomplishments

The Chair's Research Program

The CHSRF/CIHR Chair in Knowledge Transfer and Innovation program originated in research I carried out during the 1990s and derived naturally from my previous research program on science and innovation policies initiated in the 1970s. Indeed, research programs on science policy conducted until twenty years ago were more about research transfer than about science policy.

The idea that informal knowledge transfer might occur without a formal contract, as is the usual practice in technology transfer, emerged in the United States during the 1970s. Informal knowledge transfer, referred to as knowledge utilization in the United States, lost its impetus during the 1980s and 1990s, likely because it did not deliver research results from which to derive practical implications. However, these US studies on knowledge use (Frenk, 1992) enabled the re-emergence of a stronger research program on knowledge use in Canada.

My own research program and application for a CHSRF/CIHR chair award in knowledge transfer were based on these US empirical pioneering studies on knowledge use. The chair's research program has evolved over time in order to take into account changes in the research and policy environments that surround knowledge transfer. This research program led to the production of many reports prepared for policy-makers and to the publication of articles in the scholarly literature. Most of these publications were co-authored with doctoral students. One of these former doctoral students, Nabil Amara, was hired as faculty member at the department of management of Laval University. As Amara's involvement grew in preparing applications for research grants, reports, conference papers and publications, along with recruiting graduate students, he became co-director of the chair in knowledge transfer and innovation and took over many of the responsibilities of the chair's program.

The Chair's Relationships with Decision-Makers

My original application for a CHSRF/CIHR chair award also focused on the importance of building networks between researchers and users of research, especially decision- and policy-makers. This part of the overall strategy aimed at building from, and extending, my existing network of partners. The chair's formal decision-making partner was the Quebec Ministry of Health and Social Services. Early on in the partnership, the ministry created the position of knowledge transfer officer, and this officer participated on a weekly basis in various activities undertaken by the chair. At the same time, the officer was actively involved in supervising graduate students who went to the ministry as interns, usually for four-month periods. The internship program was well adapted for students enrolled in master's training programs because it provided them with opportunities to show what they were able to do. Most of these interns ended up finding jobs at the Ministry of Health and Social Services or in other ministries in the Quebec government. The program did not generate as much interest with doctoral students, who found it difficult to stop working on their research to undertake a four-month internship. Over time, it appeared more appropriate to involve doctoral students on a part-time basis at the ministry. As chair I also became involved in a concerted action with four ministries of the Quebec government (health, education, economic development, and labour) in a project on innovation in government agencies. We worked closely with an advisory committee in order to produce a systematic review and guidelines to develop a scoreboard on innovation in government agencies.

Furthermore, during the last two to three years of my chair, in dialogue with policy-makers and managers of knowledge and technology transfer organizations, many of our collaborators from the chair's program were invited to translate the findings of statistical studies and systematic reviews into knowledge transfer tools and best-practice guidelines. At the request of the Canadian Stroke Network, our team collaborated with a team based at Dalhousie University to develop a knowledge translation planning tool for biomedical researchers in stroke research, and a second tool for researchers in population health and health services doing research on stroke issues. More recently, at the request of the Quebec's Ministry of Education, Leisure and Sports, and in collaboration with representatives of schools and school boards, our team developed a knowledge transfer tool for decision-makers (school principals, pedagogic coordinators, and school boards administrators) in education. This tool is based on a systematic review of the literature on knowledge transfer in education. We initially developed a printed version with best practice guidelines on knowledge transfer. We also developed a web version of the tool, which is available on the Ministry of Education and the chair's websites. Since 2000, as the chair holder, I have frequently served as a resource on knowledge transfer in many working groups and advisory committees involved in the development of programs and activities to foster knowledge transfer.

The chair's overall strategy for networking also relied on personal contacts and opportunities provided by events, workshops, and professional conferences in which we promoted a virtual network that we created and nurtured with a short weekly electronic newsletter, *E.Watch on Innovation in Health Services*. The newsletter provides information on upcoming events, recently published reports, new or upgraded relevant websites, and subscriber-submitted events, reports, job opportunities, and so on. In 2000, fewer than 100 subscribers received the newsletter every Monday morning at 8:30 a.m. By 2009, it had more than 6,000 subscribers. Most are health professionals and policy analysts who work in health departments, regional health authorities, and other healthcare organizations in Canada and abroad. Initially, students involved in the chair's program produced the newsletter. After about sixteen months, we concluded that we needed to professionalize it, and decided to contract out its production and dissemination to three former students who created GLS Réseaux Inc. This spin-off firm on strategic intelligence currently works with many public and private organizations, in addition to producing newsletters related to public health, work and health, back injuries, genetic tests, economic development, innovation, and more. The chair's newsletter has become a template that many organizations want to replicate. Each issue is posted on the chair's website, which also provides access to knowledge transfer tools and to a weekly alert on recent scholarly articles on knowledge transfer and innovation, and which receives about half a million unique hits per year.

The Chair's Teaching Environment

The third part of the original application for a chair award related to the training of students on knowledge transfer. During the first two years, the chair was based in Laval University's Department of Political Science and had access to students enrolled in graduate programs in political science and public policy. We initially recruited and trained many students who completed master's programs and went on to work for the Quebec Ministry of Health and Social Services and for regional health authorities. Over time, many of them also seized job opportunities offered by ministries and organizations involved in economic development, innovation, agriculture, and social welfare. Other former collaborators and graduates from the chair are currently involved in the practice of knowledge transfer, working in the policy-making arena in various government agencies, at the marketing department of L'Oréal in Paris, and at the United Nations office of Dakar. One was recently elected as a member of Quebec's legislative assembly.

When the chair moved to Laval's Faculty of Business, the student pool for recruitment changed significantly. We quickly realized that most students in master's of business administration programs are neither interested in, nor trained to work on, research projects or with healthcare organizations. However, because our graduate course on evaluation methods attracted many graduate and doctoral students from the medical school, we naturally had access to a new pool of students. Furthermore, at about the same time, we also came in contact with doctoral students from the Faculty of Business who were interested in research on knowledge transfer and in working in partnership with healthcare organizations. As a consequence, our move to the Faculty of Business led us to recruit more students at the doctoral level and fewer students at the master's level. Many of these students have now completed their doctoral degrees, and former graduates from the chair are currently faculty members at various academic institutions.

Unexpectedly, our move to the Faculty of Business also significantly modified the chair's research program through teaching-related changes. Following the move, the head of the Department of Management asked me to develop a course on knowledge transfer and suggested adding "knowledge management" to its title to attract more students. During its first two years, about three-quarters of the course's content dealt with knowledge transfer and the rest with issues related to knowledge management. Over time, knowledge management became more important, and we realized that knowledge transfer research and practices needed to pay more attention to organization and management. We developed a conceptual model that integrates both perspectives, and worked with the World Health Organization on knowledge management and knowledge transfer. As an increasing number of MBA students enrolled in the course, we began to pay more attention to issues related to knowledge transfer and its counterpart, knowledge protection (e.g., patents) in private firms, in order to address their areas of interest. Two years later, I was asked to develop a doctoral course on the management of the knowledge value chain. This course provided a renewed opportunity to integrate the "knowledge transfer as a value creation process" (Landry, 2009) and three complementary perspectives – knowledge transfer, knowledge management, and value chain perspectives – into a single conceptual framework. More recently, this framework expanded to include the idea of business models.

This short history of the chair suggests that knowledge transfer, as both a field of practice and a field of research, has drastically evolved over the past twenty years. As a field of research, knowledge transfer refers to the processes by which knowledge moves from one party (the source) to another (the user or potential user). As a field of practice, knowledge transfer refers to the processes by which the knowledge of one party combines with that of another party in new or improved ways, in order to develop or improve goods, services, practices, and policies. In the rest of this chapter, we illustrate how the dialogue between policy-makers and researchers has been instrumental in the evolution of understanding what knowledge transfer is, as a research field and as a field of practice, and how to conceptually approach knowledge transfer.

From Knowledge Transfer to Knowledge Management: The Evolution of a Field

Policy-makers' growing expectations of knowledge transfer can be explained by the very large public investment in research, especially in health research, and the incapacity of many highly promising scientific results to contribute to the development or improvement of goods, services, practices, or policies. Such a context helped justify the establishment of new types of organizations, such as the Canadian Health Services Research Foundation, dedicated to promoting a more systematic implementation of research evidence into practical applications. In reaction, efforts to increase the implementation of university research have evolved as our understanding of knowledge transfer has improved. First, we present, as stage one in the development process of knowledge transfer, the traditional knowledge transfer models and their associated policy models. In stage two, we compare commercial and informal knowledge transfer. In stage three, we show that the production of research knowledge and its transfer outside the academic community are complementary.

Stage One: Traditional Knowledge Transfer Models

In most developed countries, biomedical and health sciences receive nearly half of the national research investments. The pool of biomedical research knowledge is immense and growing at a pace of roughly two million new scientific articles every year. However, a study regarding the translation of highly promising basic research into clinical applications, which screened 101 articles published in top basic science journals between 1979 and 1983, found that: "Two decades later, only 5 of these promises were in licensed clinical use and only one of them had a major impact on current medical practices. Three quarters of the basic science promises had not yet been tested in a randomized trial" (Ioannidis, 2004, p. 2). Moreover, and less reassuring, researchers from the United States and the Netherlands have estimated that 30 to 45 per cent of patients are not receiving care according to scientific evidence and that 20 to 25 per cent of the care provided is not needed or potentially harmful (Grol, 2001; McGlynn et al., 2003; Schuster et al., 1998). Clearly, expectations regarding the translation of highly promising research discoveries into practical applications are not met. This reality test has induced researchers and policy-makers to join forces to figure out ways to increase the benefits from large public and private research investments.

Until the 1970s and the rise of the knowledge transfer science-push model, policy-makers and taxpayers assumed that investments in research generated significant returns more or less automatically. This assumption was questioned and replaced by other assumptions, which led to the formulation of many other policy intervention models. The literature on policy intervention models of knowledge transfer focuses on four major alternatives (Kline & Rosenberg, 1986; Landry, 1990; Weiss, 1979; Yin & Moore, 1988): a science-push model, a demand-pull model, a dissemination model, and an interaction model. While each model supports the importance of research results in policy-making, they identify different major determinants of knowledge transfer and policy instruments to increase transfer. Alone and with colleagues from the CHSRF/CIHR Chair in Knowledge Transfer and Innovation, I contributed to this research and policy debate on several occasions (Landry, 1990; Landry et al., 2001; Landry et al., 2003).

The knowledge transfer science-push model identifies the supply of advances in research findings as the major determinant of the use of research knowledge to develop or improve products, services, and practices. In this model, researchers generate ideas for directing research and users receive the results. Transfer follows a linear sequence from supply of research advances to transmission to decision-makers and practitioners. Prior studies have considered many dimensions of research results attributes that could be influenced by policy-makers in order to increase transfer, including (1) content attributes, notably efficiency, compatibility, complexity, validity, reliability, divisibility, applicability, radicalness, and the ease of observation and trial (Dearing & Meyer, 1994; Edwards, 1991; Lomas, 1993); and (2) the type of research, such as basic/applied, general/abstract (Machlup, 1980), quantitative/qualitative (Huberman & Thurler, 1991), and particular/concrete (Rich, 1997), as well as research domains and disciplines (Oh, 1997; Rich, 1997). Empirical studies have failed to find a relationship between the technical quality of research results and transfer (Dunn, 1983; Edwards, 1991; Huberman, 1987).

The science-push conceptual model became the cornerstone for the science policy model of the 1970s. Researchers and policy-makers formulated two main critiques of this model: (1) knowledge transfer to users is not automatic in a context where no one assumes responsibility for it; and (2) untreated research results do not constitute directly usable knowledge, but should follow a transformation process to become usable in policy-making (Lomas, 1990). These criticisms have led policy-makers and researchers in science to develop a complementary model, the demand-pull model (Landry, 1990).

In the demand-pull model, which progressively emerged in the 1980s, users, rather than researchers, are the major source of ideas for directing research (Rich, 1991; Weiss, 1979; Yin & Moore, 1988). This approach generates a customer-contractor relationship in which practitioners and decision-makers behave like customers who define what research they want, and researchers behave like contractors who execute work in exchange for payment. This model also follows a linear sequence that starts with the identification of a research problem by the customers. Knowledge transfer is explained only by users' needs. It is assumed that the use of knowledge to develop or improve products, services, practices, and policies increases when policy-makers induce researchers to focus their projects on the users' needs and practical problems instead of on the advancement of scholarly knowledge (Chelimsky, 1997; Frenk, 1992; Orlandi, 1996; Silversides, 1997). However, this model does not take into account that even when research is designed to solve practical problems, results may be discarded due to potential conflicts with users' organizational interests.

The organizational interests model is a variant of the demand-pull model. It assumes that organizational structures, rules, and norms are essential determinants of knowledge transfer (Oh & Rich, 1993), and that the principal factor causing under-transfer of research material into applications lies in users' political interests, which may conflict with research findings. This perspective was considered especially relevant for policy-makers in health services, where powerful professional groups take centre stage in the management, production, and delivery of services. According to this perspective, research results are more likely to be used when they support the interests and the goals of the organization (Oh, 1997). Both the organizational interests and the demand-pull models have been criticized for: (1) focusing on the instrumental use of research and neglecting the fact that different types of knowledge lead to different uses, (2) putting too much emphasis on the users' egotistical interests, and (3) failing to consider how interactions between producers and users of research findings may increase transfer.

The knowledge transfer dissemination model was developed in the social and health services sciences in response to observations showing that, while examples of unplanned knowledge transfer existed, knowledge transfer was not automatic. This model suggests that another series of activities should be added to research projects. These activities aim to develop mechanisms to identify useful knowledge and transfer it to potential users. Dissemination occurs when a potential user becomes aware of the research results. In this model, policy-makers have two levers to improve knowledge transfer to goods, services, practices, and policies: one is the adaptation of research results for target users, and the other is the active circulation of adapted knowledge to relevant users. In many cases, the products of research are never widely spread and thus have little impact (MacLean, 1996). Policy-makers and researchers in science policy and in the research field of diffusion of innovation concluded in the 1990s that the main shortcoming of the dissemination model was that the potential users are not involved in the selection of the transferable information or in the production of research results.

The knowledge transfer interaction model was developed in the 1990s to overcome shortcomings of the previous models (Dunn, 1980; Huberman & Thurler, 1991; Nyden & Wiewel, 1992; Oh, 1997; Yin & Moore, 1988) and was the model initially adopted by CHSRF. The interaction model suggests that knowledge transfer into applicable contexts depends on various disorderly interactions that occur between researchers and users, rather than on linear sequences that begin with the researchers' or users' needs.

The interaction model combines the explanatory factors and the policy instruments identified in prior models. It suggests four areas of action to increase transfer: (1) types of research and scientific disciplines, (2) needs and organizational interests of users, (3) dissemination processes, and (4) linkage mechanisms between researchers and users. The initial empirical studies conducted by Landry, Amara, and collaborators were based on models from this first phase. Although these early conceptual models are still largely used in researchers' and policy-makers' communities, the emerging debate in knowledge transfer suggests the need to pay more attention to the role of organizational processes in transforming research knowledge into practical applications, and to the contribution of research knowledge into the development or improvement of goods, services, practices, and policies.

To sum up, changes in our understanding of how research transfer works paved the way to two overlapping research programs: one that deals with the transfer of technologies, and a second one that deals with the transfer of knowledge spillovers.

Stage Two: Transfer through Commercialization of Knowledge versus Transfer of Knowledge Spillovers

Over recent decades, universities have become increasingly involved in technology transfer through the establishment of technology transfer offices, technology licensing, business incubators, technology parks, and venture capital funds for start-up companies. The field of health services research has not stimulated the emergence of equivalent institutions, and knowledge transfer was left to the initiatives of individual researchers. The creation of CHSRF was instrumental in filling this void and Jonathan Lomas, its inaugural CEO, advocated for the importance of paying attention to the transfer and implementation of research evidence into health services.

Scholarly studies on research transfer have primarily concentrated on the commercialization of research and the protection of intellectual property. Knowledge transfer between universities and industry or government agencies has been tracked through patent data (Hall & Ziedonis, 2001; Henderson et al., 1998; Mowery et al., 2002), citation analyses (Spencer, 2001), licensing (Jensen & Thursby, 2001; Thursby & Thursby, 2002, 2003), spin-off creations (Link & Scott, 2005; O'Shea et al., 2005; Powers & McDougall, 2005; Shane & Stuart, 2002; Zucker et al., 2002), collaboration between universities and industry and/or government agencies (Cohen et al., 2002; Irwin et al., 1998; Lee, 1996; Owen-Smith et al., 2002; D'Este & Patel, 2005), and assessing university technology transfer offices (Rogers et al., 2000; Trune & Goslin, 1998).

A Statistics Canada survey on the commercialization of intellectual property in universities (Read, 2005) shows that, in 2003, Canadian researchers based in universities reported 1,133 inventions, filed 1,252 patent applications, and helped to create 64 spin-off companies. The income generated from intellectual property amounted to $55.5 million and universities spent a total of $36.4 million for intellectual property management. In 2006, research investments in Canadian universities amounted to $10.4 billion (AUCC, 2008). These figures suggest very low returns on investments: $10.4 billion invested to generate an income of $55.5 million, minus $36.4 million in operational expenditures. These results carry two implications: either investments in university research do not generate acceptable returns, or indicators used to measure returns on investments (such as patents, licenses, and spinoffs) are not valid.

If the indicators are insufficient, there is a need for research on other mechanisms that can transmit knowledge spillovers. Knowledge spillovers transmitted through university researchers refer to when people based in firms, government agencies, and other organizations access knowledge from university researchers but do not fully compensate them (Audretsch et al., 2004; Harris, 2001; Landry et al., 2007). Studies on the mechanisms behind such transfers are scanty. We will now consider mechanisms of knowledge transfer that involve knowledge spillovers, and how often and when they are used. Over the past ten years, the chair has focused most of its activities on the transfer of knowledge spillovers through various formal and informal mechanisms. My chair program's contribution in this respect relates to the development of validated scales of knowledge transfer and knowledge use, and to the training of graduate students in this subfield of knowledge transfer.

Technology transfer is a construct that refers to the instrumentality of knowledge; sets of tangible tools stored in blueprints, databases, manuals, and other forms of documents, such as patents. These attributes transform technology into products that are easily amenable to commercial transactions. However, knowledge in health services can be more tacit, less tangible, and embodied in theories and principles regarding cause-and-effect relationships that are stored in people's heads. These attributes of knowledge suggest the use of a process approach to conceptualization and operationalization of knowledge spillovers. In this approach, researchers identify how the knowledge produced across the different stages of research moves into the various decision-making activities of the recipients (Landry, Amara, & Lamari, 2001; Landry, Lamari, & Amara, 2003; Lomas, 1997). Assuming that a discrete decision can be attributed to the use of a single study is too simplistic: research findings have many effects (Mandell & Sauter, 1984), and decisions do not usually depend on a single study but rather on a series of syntheses that converge in one direction (Booth, 1990; Lomas, 1997; Rich, 1997). Therefore, the transfer of knowledge spillovers should be conceptualized and implemented as a series of activities that feed decision-making, such as transmission of research results, presentation of research results, participation in working groups involving users, and contribution to the development of goods or services.

Research findings on the transfer of knowledge spillovers (Landry et al., 2001, 2007) show that university researchers were active in the transfer of their knowledge, even when they did not receive financial compensation for the results of their work. Furthermore, increases in knowledge transfer are related to increases in the number of publications, which suggests that the second activity does not jeopardize the first.

These findings (Landry et al., 2001, 2007) are interesting for other reasons. We gathered statistical evidence that indicates that researchers in certain research fields were much more active in knowledge transfer than those in others. We also obtained evidence that shows that only two factors are associated with variations in knowledge transfer activities throughout all research fields: (1) linkages between researchers and users and (2) the focus of research projects on users' needs.

These results have some practical implications for policy-makers. First, given the frequency of non-commercial knowledge transfer, policy-makers should pay more attention to knowledge transfer that does not involve the commercialization of protected intellectual property. Consequently, university technology transfer offices can or should revise their mandates to create opportunities to share non-commercial knowledge for research disciplines related to social sciences and health services research. Second, universal policies intended to foster knowledge transfer should take into account the fact that only a limited number of predictors significantly explain transfer variations across research fields. Third, in addition to universal policy measures, customized measures should be developed to increase knowledge transfer, given that certain factors contribute to an increased transfer only in specific research fields. Our research (Landry et al., 2007) shows that knowledge transfer cannot be reduced to simply forging better links between researchers and research users. Contingent factors that are difficult to integrate into general theories also influence knowledge transfer.

At the beginning of the 2000s, researchers in knowledge transfer and leading policy-makers developed a renewed understanding of knowledge transfer base. Two types of evidence fuelled this activity. First, the linkage model of knowledge transfer, which focuses on the exchange of knowledge between individual researchers and individual users, appeared to be insufficient and had to be complemented by taking into account the role of organizational processes in knowledge management within and between organizations. Second, empirical research did not corroborate the postulated potential conflict between advancing knowledge through publications and forging links between researchers and users. Many researchers started to investigate complementarities between publications and various forms of knowledge transfer.

This new understanding led researchers and policy-makers to abandon linear views of knowledge transfer. Instead, they began to associate knowledge transfer with processes in which the knowledge of one party is combined with the knowledge of another party to develop or improve goods, services, practices, and policies. This revised view led to studies on complementarities between academic activities and to the development of knowledge management initiatives.

Stage Three: Complementarities between Academic Activities

The persistent perception that university research is under-used has led many policy-makers to assume that university researchers maximize publications at the expense of knowledge transfer to users outside the academic community. When considering the performance effects of differences in resources that academics invest in different activities, two hypotheses emerge: the substitution and the complementary hypotheses (Colbeck, 1998; Mitchell & Rebne, 1995; Walckiers, 2004). The substitution hypothesis, which is the dominating view in policy circles, rests on the idea that academics are resource-constrained, and so investments in one academic activity, such as publishing in academic journals, are made at the expense of investments and performance in other activities, such as sharing research results with users in health services organizations (Mitchell & Rebne, 1995; Walckiers, 2004). This hypothesis assumes academic researchers divide their resources unequally and concentrate on activities for which they are the most productive. The substitution hypothesis implicitly assumes that academic activities are separate, dissociated, and fragmented, and that resources invested in one activity are resources not invested in others (Colbeck, 1998).

The complementary hypothesis suggests that resources invested in one academic activity predict performance in both that activity and also in associated activities (Mitchell & Rebne, 1995; Walckiers, 2004). Each academic activity generates ideas that become inputs for other activities. More concretely, the outputs of certain academic activities may become asset bases upon which other academic activities are built. As a consequence, performance in certain academic activities may generate a leverage effect on others. The complementary hypothesis is recurring in the literature on academic activities, as exhibited by the following claims:

- "Being active in research might improve teaching skills and vice versa" (Walckiers, 2004, p. 3);
- Teaching and research activities cannot be dissociated (Colbeck, 1998; Layzell, 1996; Walckiers, 2004);
- Teaching and research merge in a "seamless blend" (Clark, 1987, p. 70);
- The increase in interactions between science and technology suggests that certain academic activities may be complementary (Azoulay et al., 2006; Etzkowitz & Leydesdorff, 1997; Gibbons et al., 1994; Narin et al., 1997);
- The triple helix model of knowledge exchange between university, industry, and government also points to the idea that research, knowledge, and technology transfer activities may be complementary (Etzkowitz, 2003; Etzkowitz & Leydesdorff, 1997; Etzkowitz et al., 1998; Gibbons et al., 1994).

In response to such concerns, with other collaborators from the CHSRF/CIHR Chair in Knowledge Transfer and Innovation (Landry, Saïhi, Amara, & Ouimet, 2010), we explored whether six academic activities – teaching, publishing, patenting, spin-off creation, consulting, and producing knowledge spillovers – are complementary, substitute, or in conflict. Consistent with many prior studies that indicated the presence of complementarities between pairs of activities such as publications and patenting, our results suggest that publishing, patenting, spin-off creation, consulting, and producing knowledge spillovers are complementary. These factors are interdependent and reinforce one other, and so to improve understanding and science policies, we should approach these activities jointly.

However, contrary to many claims (Colbeck, 1998; Walckiers, 2004), our results also suggest that teaching and publishing are exclusive activities. Increased teaching occurs at the expense of publication, and vice versa. Again, this result carries implications for our understanding and for the management of universities, at the level of both individual academic careers and also institutional managers and policy-makers, who should approach these activities independently rather than as joint activities that reinforce and consolidate each other.

Surprisingly, our results did not support the substitution hypothesis between teaching and patenting, spin-off creation, consulting, and producing knowledge spillovers. Instead, we found independence between them. This result implies that patenting, spin-off creation, consulting, and producing knowledge spillovers have neither positive nor adverse effects on teaching.

Overall, our results suggest the existence of three very different types of academic portfolios. A first portfolio is made up of complementary activities that are interdependent and reinforce each other. This portfolio includes publishing, patenting, spin-off creation, consulting, and producing. A second portfolio includes teaching and publishing, which are substitutes for each other. A third portfolio includes teaching and activities independent from teaching, namely, patenting, spin-off creation, consulting, and producing knowledge spillovers. The results of our study suggest that complementary activities may facilitate entry to and successful performance in other activities, while substitute activities may hamper entry to and performance in specific other activities. See Siggelkow (2002) and Stieglitz and Heine (2007) for a detailed discussion on complementarities and substitution in organizations.

Knowledge Management

At the beginning of the twenty-first century, policy-makers in large organizations – especially in healthcare organizations and in public health organizations like the World Health Organization – came to think that focusing attention on individuals and linkages between them would not sufficiently increase knowledge transfer. Recall that most knowledge transfer policy interventions tend to focus on individual researchers (as sources of knowledge) and individual users (as potential consumers of knowledge), as well as on the individual resources and attributes that are likely to influence knowledge transfer and uptake. By comparison, knowledge management studies tend to focus on organizations and how organizational resources and characteristics affect knowledge transfer and implementation in the development or improvement of goods, services, or organizational practices.

In the management literature, knowledge is the resource with the highest strategic value for organizations. The ability to acquire, create, share, and apply knowledge represents organizations' most significant capacity to solve health services problems. Two characteristics arise from such a perspective: the first relates to the process nature of knowledge application, the second to the aim of knowledge application, which is to create value for organizations. These two characteristics suggest that knowledge should be managed and used to add value to the production and delivery processes of health services organizations. In the management literature, this idea of value creation is often approached through the concept of the knowledge value chain.

In response to this new emerging concern, I, along with collaborators from the World Health Organization and CHSRF, developed a knowledge value chain framework organized around five dyadic capabilities that support the concept of the chain in public health organizations. There is no consensus on the critical capabilities required to manage knowledge productively (Holsapple & Joshi, 2002). However, five dyadic capabilities appear to be important: (1) mapping and acquisition complement each other; (2) creation is partly associated with destruction; (3) integration depends on sharing and transfer; (4) replication relates to protection; and (5) performance assessment is linked to innovation. Knowledge creation is the capability that has received the most attention in the research community. The others are less documented, but the management literature has something to say about each of them.

From an organizational perspective, the interdependence of such dyadic capabilities generates a value chain that moves from knowledge mapping and acquisition up to the production and delivery of new or improved public health programs and interventions, which results in added value for people (Holsapple & Singh, 2001; Lee & Yang, 2000; Lundquist, 2003). The mission, vision, goals, and strategies of a public health organization or social enterprise drive the knowledge value chain. The higher the knowledge performance related to dyadic capabilities, the more value is generated.

Knowledge Mapping and Knowledge Acquisition

Internal knowledge mapping involves the ability of public health organizations to know what they know. It refers to an organization's understanding and self-awareness of its knowledge resources and their limitations (Spinello, 1998). Internal knowledge is especially important because it is unique, specific to the organization, and tacit – and

Figure 3.1 The Knowledge Value Chain

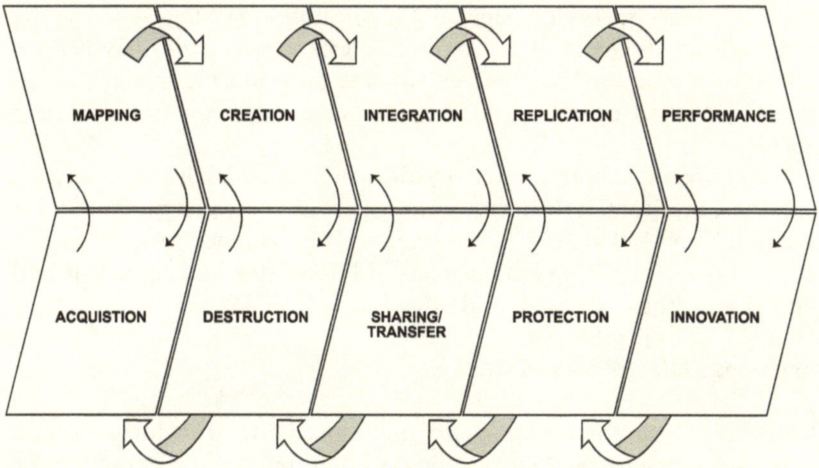

therefore difficult for external knowledge holders to reproduce. External knowledge acquisition refers to an organization's ability to identify and acquire information from outside sources and make it suitable for subsequent use. Knowledge mapping and acquisition involve many more specific capacities, such as locating, accessing, valuing, and filtering pertinent knowledge; extracting, collecting, distilling, refining, interpreting, packaging, and transforming it into usable knowledge; and moving the usable knowledge within the organization for subsequent use in problem-solving activities (Holsapple & Joshi, 2002). External knowledge may provide new ideas and context for benchmarking internal knowledge; this external knowledge is more explicit and more costly to acquire, but easily available to other organizations.

Knowledge Creation and Destruction

The size of internal and external knowledge gaps influences knowledge creation. The knowledge creation capability refers to the capacity to combine knowledge with knowledge (tacit and explicit, individual and collective, internal and external), as well as with other resources, in order to develop new intelligence to produce and deliver better public health outputs and outcomes (Nonaka & Takeuchi, 1995; Nonaka &

Toyama, 2005). Knowledge creation is usually associated with research and development activities. However, it should also include activities such as problem solving, devising a promotion strategy, discovering a pattern, or developing a program or intervention, all of which can apply to public health. Needless to say, only individuals can create knowledge, but organizations support and amplify it (Lee & Yang, 2000).

We know little about knowledge destruction, which is the capacity to eliminate or disentangle the interconnectedness between pieces of information (Kaplan et al., 2001). The literature on evidence-based medicine shows how difficult it is to destroy old knowledge and replace it with new (for example, clinical guidelines).

Knowledge Integration and Transfer

Knowledge integration refers to the capacity to transform existing knowledge resources (tacit, explicit, individual, organizational, internal, external, and created knowledge) into actionable knowledge by taking into account the strengths, weaknesses, opportunities, and threats that face a public health organization (Lee & Yang, 2000). Over time, public health organizations develop more or less explicit processes to synthesize the internal knowledge accumulated over time with that acquired from other external sources (such as other organizations, scientific publications, or clinical guidelines).

Integrating disjointed pieces of raw knowledge into actionable knowledge is necessary but not sufficient. Knowledge must also be shared and transferred in order to help solve public health problems. Knowledge sharing makes pertinent information available to others within an organization, program, project, or intervention (Ipe, 2003). Knowledge sharing is more demanding than knowledge reporting (Davenport, 1997). Reporting involves dissemination of information into codified formats (your information technology system) to target groups within a public health organization. By contrast, sharing involves person-to-person interactions where one individual converts (individual and often tacit) knowledge into a form that other members in the organization can understand (Hendriks, 1999). Knowledge sharing is the mechanism by which individual knowledge can be transformed into organizational knowledge, which then can be redeployed to create value and solve problems at the organizational level. In addition, knowledge sharing is a social process that may lead to the emergence of communities of practice (Wenger et al., 2002). In public health, such communities exist at the local, regional, national, and international levels. Knowledge transfer complements knowledge sharing.

Knowledge Replication and Protection

Knowledge that has been shared or transferred provides a template or a guideline for decisions and actions. Knowledge replication involves identifying the attributes, methods, and contexts necessary for successful recreation (Winter & Szulanski, 2001). Replicating templates and guidelines is never easy. There are always significant differences between the attributes of the knowledge and the context of action and decision described in templates and guidelines on the one hand, and a real public health context on the other. Moreover, shared and transferred knowledge does not come with a how-to manual appropriate to any local conditions. The many idiosyncratic features of the local contexts in which public health organizations operate make precisely replicating templates and guidelines difficult, if not impossible. Knowledge replication must be guided by the attributes of the local context of actions and decisions, especially with respect to public health.

The capacity to replicate knowledge improves the efficacy and efficiency of public health programs and interventions. However, knowledge protection limits knowledge replication through legal mechanisms, such as patents, copyrights, trademarks, and confidentiality agreements. Public health organizations aim to facilitate knowledge replications in a context where the biomedical industry frequently emphasizes knowledge protection (i.e., patent protection).

Knowledge Performance and Innovation

Knowledge performance is the capacity to assess the extent to which knowledge replication delivers the desired outcomes. Assessments are usually undertaken for one or a combination of four perspectives that aim to balance the financial and non-financial outcomes (Carlucci, Marr et al., 2004): (1) the value for money, or the public health benefits derived from investments into knowledge creation, sharing, and application; (2) knowledge users' means to assess the extent to which public health policy decisions, community initiatives, and professional practices are based on sound evidence, and to assess the extent to which evidence-based policy decisions and evidence-based professional practices contribute to developing or improving products and services; (3) the final beneficiaries of knowledge translation, or the extent to which evidence-based policy decisions and professional practices translate into new or improved products and services, and superior public health outcomes thereof; and (4) the internal organizational process, which aims to provide an account of the activities organizations must develop and excel at to achieve a superior knowledge creation, sharing, transfer, and replication milieu for evidence-based policy decisions and professional practices, and to achieve superior outcomes for the final beneficiaries of knowledge application.

Conclusion: Knowledge Transfer as a Value Creation Process

Knowledge transfer and knowledge management are increasingly considered incomplete, and a growing number of advocates call for the development of the more comprehensive concept of knowledge transfer as a value creation process (Landry, 2009). Such a perspective transforms the traditional problem of increasing knowledge transfer into the problem of creating or increasing value from the use of knowledge.

Much of the literature on technology transfer focuses on knowledge creation (research and publications) and the appropriation of the returns of research knowledge (patents, licenses, spin-off creation, service innovations, practice innovations, and policy innovations). This stream of knowledge transfer studies considers research knowledge a mature object that can be directly observed, stored, and transferred for use and reuse (Albino et al., 2004; Landry et al., 2007; Szulanski, 2000). Likewise, much of the literature on knowledge translation focuses on building interactions between researchers and users, and on adapting and disseminating research knowledge for users. This second stream of studies also implicitly considers research knowledge a mature object that is underused because of communication problems between researchers and users. Recent studies by Landry (2009) and others contend that both these approaches to knowledge transfer underestimate the immature character of scientific promises, and also underestimate the importance of the transformation process of raw research knowledge into new or improved products, services, practices, or policies. In the coming years, there will be a rise in the number of studies focusing on the capability of organizations to acquire, create, share, and apply knowledge to improve services and practices regarding healthcare problems (Landry et al., 2006). This hypotheses rests on the idea that organizations that rely on research knowledge to innovate (that is, to develop or improve policies, programs, interventions, and professional practices) have superior knowledge transformation processes (English & Baker, 2006, p. 98).

In the 1990s, Canadian scholars played an important role in the re-emergence of the knowledge use field, later renamed knowledge translation by CIHR and CHSRF. The field was initially dominated by reflexive and conceptual pieces and case studies that adopted the individual as the unit of analysis and the target of policy interventions. The work of Canadian scholars promoted the evidence-based decision-making movement in Canadian healthcare organizations. By comparison, our chair implemented a quantitative research program on knowledge transfer, while moving progressively from reliance on the individual towards the adoption of the organization as a unit of analysis and target of intervention.

REFERENCES

Albino, V., Garavelli, A.C., & Gorgoglione, M. (2004). Organization and technology in knowledge transfer. *Benchmarking: An International Journal, 11*(6), 584–600. http://dx.doi.org/10.1108/14635770410566492

AUCC. (2008). *En plein essor, edition 2008 du rapport sur la recherché universitaire et la mobilisation du savoir.* Ottawa: AUCC.

Audretsch, D.B., Lehmann, E.E., & Warning, S. (2004). University spillovers: Does the kind of science matter? *Industry and Innovation, 11*(3), 193–206. http://dx.doi.org/10.1080/1366271042000265375

Azoulay, P., Ding, W., & Stuart, T. (2006). *The impact of academic patenting on the rate, quality, and direction of (public) research output.* NBER Working Paper No. 11917, January 2006.

Booth, T. (1990). Researching policy research. *Knowledge-Creation Diffusion Utilization, 12*(1), 80–100.

Carlucci, D., Marr, B., & Schiuma, G. (2004). The knowledge value chain: How intellectual capital impacts on business performance. *International Journal of Technology Management, 27*(6/7), 575–88. http://dx.doi.org/10.1504/IJTM.2004.004903

Chelimsky, E. (1997). The coming transformation in evaluation. In E. Chelimsky & W.R. Shadish (Eds.), *Evaluation for the 21st century* (pp. 45–62). Thousand Oaks, CA: Sage Publications.

Clark, B.R. (1987). *The academic life: Small worlds, different worlds*. Princeton, NJ: Carnegie Foundation for the Advancement of Teaching.

Cohen, W.M., Nelson, R.R., & Walsh, J.P. (2002). Links and impacts: The influence of public research on industrial R&D. *Management Science, 48*(1), 1–23. http://dx.doi.org/10.1287/mnsc.48.1.1.14273

Colbeck, C.L. (1998). Merging in a seamless blend. How faculty integrate teaching and research. *Journal of Higher Education, 69*(6), 647–71. http://dx.doi.org/10.2307/2649212

Davenport, T.H. (1997). *Information ecology*. Oxford, UK: Oxford University Press.

Dearing, J.W., & Meyer, G. (1994). An exploratory tool for predicting adoption decisions. *Science Communication, 16*(1), 43–57. http://dx.doi.org/10.1177/0164025994016001003

D'Este, P., & Patel, P. (2005). University-industry linkages in the UK: What are the factors determining the variety of interactions with industry. In Proceedings of 5th Triple Helix Conference, Turin, Italy, 18–21 May.

Dunn, W.N. (1980). The two communities metaphor and models of knowledge use. *Knowledge-Creation Diffusion Utilization, 1*, 515–36.

Dunn, W.N. (1983). Measuring knowledge use. *Knowledge-Creation Diffusion Utilization, 5*(1), 120–33.

Edwards, L.A. (1991). *Using knowledge and technology to improve the quality of life of people who have disabilities: A prosumer approach*. Philadelphia, PA: Knowledge Utilization Program, Pennsylvania College of Optometry.

English, M.J., & Baker, W.H., Jr. (2006). *Winning the knowledge transfer race*. New York: McGraw-Hill.

Etzkowitz, H. (2003). Innovation in innovation: The triple helix of university-industry-government relation. *Social Sciences Information. Information Sur les Sciences Sociales, 42*(3), 293–337. http://dx.doi.org/10.1177/05390184030423002

Etzkowitz, H., & Leydesdorff, L. (1997). *Universities and the global knowledge economy: A triple helix of university-industry-government relations*. London: Pinter.

Etzkowitz, H., Webster, A., & Healey, P. (1998). *Capitalizing knowledge: New intersections of industry and academia*. Albany: State University of New York Press.

Frenk, J. (1992). Balancing relevance and excellence: Organizational responses to link research with decision making. *Social Science & Medicine, 35*(11), 1397–404. http://dx.doi.org/10.1016/0277-9536(92)90043-P Medline:1462179

Gibbons, M., Limoges, C., Nowotny, H., Schwartzman, S., Scott, P., & Trow, M. (1994). *The new production of knowledge. The dynamics of science and research in contemporary societies*. London: Sage Publications.

Grol, R. (2001). Successes and failures in the implementation of evidence-based guidelines for clinical practice. *Medical Care, 39*(8), 1146–54. http://dx.doi.org/10.1097/00005650-200108002-00003 Medline:11606869

Hall, B.H., & Ziedonis, R.H. (2001). The patent paradox revisited: An empirical study of patenting in the U.S. semiconductor industry, 1979–1995. *Rand Journal of Economics, 32*(1), 101–28. http://dx.doi.org/10.2307/2696400

Harris, R.G. (2001). The knowledge-based economy: Intellectual origins and new economic perspectives. *International Journal of Management Reviews, 3*(1), 21–40. http://dx.doi.org/10.1111/1468-2370.00052

Henderson, R., Jaffe, A.B., & Trajtenberg, M. (1998). Universities as a source of commercial technology: A detailed analysis of university patenting, 1965–1988. *Review of Economics and Statistics, 80*(1), 119–27. http://dx.doi.org/10.1162/003465398557221

Hendriks, P. (1999). Why share knowledge? The influence of ICT on the motivation for knowledge sharing. *Knowledge and Process Management, 6*(2), 91–100. http://dx.doi.org/10.1002/(SICI)1099-1441(199906)6:2<91::AID-KPM54>3.0.CO;2-M

Holsapple, C.W., & Joshi, K.D. (2002). Knowledge manipulation activities: Results of a Delphi study. *Information & Management, 39*(6), 477–90. http://dx.doi.org/10.1016/S0378-7206(01)00109-4

Holsapple, C.W., & Singh, M. (2001). The knowledge chain model: Activities of competitiveness. *Expert Systems with Applications, 20*(1), 77–98. http://dx.doi.org/10.1016/S0957-4174(00)00050-6

Huberman, M. (1987). Steps toward an integrated model of research utilization. *Knowledge, 8*, 586–611.

Huberman, M., & Thurler, G. (1991). *De la recherche à la pratique. Éléments de base*. Berne: Peter Lang SA, Éditions scientifiques européennes.

Ioannidis, J.P.A. (2004). Materializing research promises: Opportunities, priorities and conflicts in translational medicine. *Journal of Translational Medicine, 2*(5), 1–6. Medline:14720299

Ipe, M. (2003). Knowledge sharing in organizations: A conceptual framework. *Human Resource Development Review, 2*(4), 337–59. http://dx.doi.org/10.1177/1534484303257985

Irwin, H., More, E., & McGrath, M. (1998). Relationship management for innovation: The central role of communication in Australia's participation in two hi-tech industries. *Technology Analysis and Strategic Management, 10*(4), 467–81. http://dx.doi.org/10.1080/09537329808524328

Jensen, R.A., & Thursby, M.C. (2001). Proofs and prototypes for sale: The tale of university licensing. *American Economic Review, 91*(1), 240–59. http://dx.doi.org/10.1257/aer.91.1.240

Kaplan, S., et al. (2001). *Knowledge-based theories of the firm in strategic management: A review and extension.* Cambridge, MA: Massachusetts Institute of Technology.

Kline, S.J., & Rosenberg, N. (1986). An overview of innovation. In R. Landau & N. Rosenberg (Eds.), *The positive sum strategy: Harnessing technology for economic growth* (pp. 275–306). Washington, DC: National Academy Press.

Landry, R. (1990). Barriers to efficient monitoring of science, technology and innovation through public policy. *Journal of Science and Public Policy, 16*(6), 345–52.

Landry, R., Saïhi, M., Amara, N., & Ouimet, M. (2010). Evidence on how academics manage their portfolio of knowledge transfer activities. *Research Policy, 39*(10), 1387–403. http://dx.doi.org/10.1016/j.respol.2010.08.003

Landry, R. (2009). Knowledge management and commercialization. In H. Straus, J. Tetroe, and I.D. Graham (Eds.), *Knowledge translation in health care: Moving from evidence to practice* (pp. 280–90). Oxford, Wiley-Blackwell, MMJ Books. http://dx.doi.org/10.1002/9781444311747.app2

Landry, R., Amara, N., & Lamari, M. (2001). Utilization of social science research knowledge in Canada. *Research Policy, 30*(2), 333–49. http://dx.doi.org/10.1016/S0048-7333(00)00081-0

Landry, R., Amara, N., & Ouimet, M. (2007). Determinants of knowledge transfer: Evidence from Canadian university researchers in natural sciences and engineering. *Journal of Technology Transfer, 32*(6), 561–92. http://dx.doi.org/10.1007/s10961-006-0017-5

Landry, R., Amara, N., Pablos-Mendes, A., Shademani, R., & Gold, I. (2006). The knowledge-value chain: A conceptual framework for knowledge translation in health. *Bulletin of the World Health Organization, 84*(8), 597–602. http://dx.doi.org/10.2471/BLT.06.031724 Medline:16917645

Landry, R., Lamari, M., & Amara, N. (2003). Extent and determinants of utilization of university research in government agencies. *Public Administration Review, 63*(2), 192–204. http://dx.doi.org/10.1111/1540-6210.00279

Layzell, D.T. (1996). Faculty workload and productivity: Recurrent issues with new imperatives. *Review of Higher Education, 19*(3), 267–82.

Lee, C.C., & Yang, J. (2000). Knowledge value chain. *Journal of Management Development, 19*(9), 783–94. http://dx.doi.org/10.1108/02621710010378228

Lee, Y.S. (1996). Technology transfer and the research university: A search for the boundaries of university-industry collaboration. *Research Policy, 25*(6), 843–63. http://dx.doi.org/10.1016/0048-7333(95)00857-8

Link, A.N., & Scott, J.T. (2005). Opening the ivory tower's door: An analysis of the determinants of the formation of U.S. university spin-off companies. *Research Policy, 34*(7), 1106–12. http://dx.doi.org/10.1016/j.respol.2005.05.015

Lomas, J. (1990). Finding audiences, changing beliefs: The structure of research use in Canadian health policy. *Journal of Health Politics, Policy and Law, 15*(3), 525–42. http://dx.doi.org/10.1215/03616878-15-3-525 Medline:2273216

Lomas, J. (1993). Diffusion, dissemination, and implementation: Who should do what? *Annals of the New York Academy of Sciences, 703*(1), 226–37. http://dx.doi.org/10.1111/j.1749-6632.1993.tb26351.x Medline: 8192299

Lomas, J. (1997). Research and evidence-based decision making. *Australian and New Zealand Journal of Public Health, 21*(5), 439–41. http://dx.doi.org/10.1111/j.1467-842X.1997.tb01730.x Medline:9343883

Lundquist, G. (2003). A rich vision of technology transfer: Technology value management. *Journal of Technology Transfer, 28*(3/4), 265–84. http://dx.doi.org/10.1023/A:1024949029313

Machlup, F. (1980). *Knowledge and knowledge production*. Princeton: Princeton Press.

MacLean, D.R. (1996). Positioning dissemination in public health policy. *Canadian Journal of Public Health, 87*(2), 40–3.

Mandell, M.B., & Sauter, V.L. (1984). Approaches to the study of information utilization in public agencies. *Journal of Knowledge-Creation, Diffusion, Utilization, 6*(2), 145–63.

McGlynn, E.A., Asch, S.M., Adams, J., Keesey, J., Hicks, J., DeCristofaro, A., & Kerr, E.A. (2003). The quality of health care delivered to adults in the United States. *The New England Journal of Medicine, 348*(26), 2635–45. http://dx.doi.org/10.1056/NEJMsa022615 Medline:12826639

Mitchell, J.E., & Rebne, D.S. (1995). The nonlinear effects of teaching and consulting on academic research productivity. *Socio-Economic Planning Sciences, 29*(1), 47–57. http://dx.doi.org/10.1016/0038-0121(95)98606-V

Mowery, D.C., Sampat, B.N., & Ziedonis, A.A. (2002). Learning to patent: Institutional experience, learning, and the characteristics of US university patents after the Bayh-Dole Act, 1981–1992. *Management Science, 48*(1), 73–89. http://dx.doi.org/10.1287/mnsc.48.1.73.14278

Narin, F., Hamilton, K., & Olivastro, D. (1997). The increasing linkage between US technology and public science. *Research Policy, 26*(3), 317–30. http://dx.doi.org/10.1016/S0048-7333(97)00013-9

Nonaka, I., & Takeuchi, H. (1995). *The knowledge-creating company: How Japanese companies create the dynamics of innovation*. New York: Oxford University Press.

Nonaka, I., & Toyama, R. (2005). The theory of the knowledge-creating firm: Subjectivity, objectivity and synthesis. *Industrial and Corporate Change, 14*(3), 419–36. http://dx.doi.org/10.1093/icc/dth058

Nyden, P., & Wiewel, W. (1992). Collaborative research: Harnessing the tensions between researchers and practitioners. *American Sociologist, 23*(4), 43–55. http://dx.doi.org/10.1007/BF02691930

Oh, C.H. (1997). Issues for new thinking of knowledge utilization: Introductory remarks. Knowledge and policy. *International Journal of Knowledge Transfer and Utilization, 10*(3), 3–10.

Oh, C.H., & Rich, R.F. (1996). Explaining use of information in public policymaking. *Knowledge and Policy, 9*(1), 3–35. http://dx.doi.org/10.1007/BF02832231

Orlandi, M. (1996). Health promotion technology transfer: Organizational perspectives. *Canadian Journal of Public Health, 87*(2), 28–33.

O'Shea, R.P., Allen, T.J., Chevalier, A., & Roche, F. (2005). Entrepreneurial orientation, technology transfer, and spinoff performance of US universities. *Research Policy, 34*(7), 994–1009. http://dx.doi.org/10.1016/j.respol.2005.05.011

Owen-Smith, J., Riccaboni, M., Pammolli, F., & Powell, W.W. (2002). A comparison of US and European university-industry relations in the life sciences. *Management Science, 48*(1), 24–43. http://dx.doi.org/10.1287/mnsc.48.1.24.14275

Powers, J.B., & McDougall, P.P. (2005). University start-up formation and technology licensing with firms that go public: A resource-based view of academic entrepreneurship. *Journal of Business Venturing, 20*(3), 291–311. http://dx.doi.org/10.1016/j.jbusvent.2003.12.008

Read, C. (2005). Survey of intellectual property commercialization in the higher education sector, 2003. Ottawa: Statistics Canada, Working Paper (88F0006XIE, 18).

Rich, R.F. (1991). Knowledge creation, dissemination, and utilization. *International Journal of Knowledge Transfer and Utilization, 12*(3), 319–37.

Rich, R.F. (1997). Measuring knowledge utilization process and outcomes. Knowledge and policy. *International Journal of Knowledge Transfer and Utilization, 10*(3), 3–10.

Rich, R.F., & Oh, C.H. (1993). The utilization of policy research. In S. Nagel (Ed.), *Encyclopedia of policy studies* (2nd ed.) (pp. 93–111). New York: Marcel Dekkar Inc.

Rogers, E., Yin, J., & Hoffmann, J. (2000). Assessing the effectiveness of technology transfer offices at US research universities. *Journal of the Association of University Technology Managers, 12*, 47–80.

Schuster, M.A., McGlynn, E.A., & Brook, R.H. (1998). How good is the quality of health care in the United States? *The Milbank Quarterly, 76*(4), 509, 517–63. http://dx.doi.org/10.1111/1468-0009.00105 Medline:9879302

Shane, S., & Stuart, T. (2002). Organizational endowments and the performance of university startups. *Management Science, 48*(1), 154–70. http://dx.doi.org/10.1287/mnsc.48.1.154.14280

Siggelkow, N. (2002). Misperceiving interactions among complements and substitutes: Organizational consequences. *Management Science, 48*(7), 900–16. http://dx.doi.org/10.1287/mnsc.48.7.900.2820

Silversides, A. (1997). Dissemination of research results to clinicians an art in itself. *Canadian Medical Association Journal, 156*(12), 1746–7. Medline:9220930

Spencer, J. (2001). How relevant is university-based scientific research to private high-technology firms? A United States-Japan comparison. *Academy of Management Journal, 44*(2), 432–40. http://dx.doi.org/10.2307/3069465

Spinello, R.A. (1998). The knowledge chain. *Business Horizons, 41*(6), 4–14. http://dx.doi.org/10.1016/S0007-6813(98)90017-9

Stieglitz, N., & Heine, K. (2007). Innovations and the role of complementarities in a strategic theory of the firm. *Strategic Management Journal, 28*(1), 1–15. http://dx.doi.org/10.1002/smj.565

Szulanski, G. (2000). The process of knowledge transfer: A diachronic analysis of stickiness. *Organizational Behavior and Human Decision Processes, 82*(1), 9–27. http://dx.doi.org/10.1006/obhd.2000.2884

Thursby, J.G., & Thursby, M.C. (2002). Who is selling the ivory tower? Sources of growth in university licensing. *Management Science, 48*(1), 90–104. http://dx.doi.org/10.1287/mnsc.48.1.90.14271

Thursby, J.G., & Thursby, M.C. (2003). Patterns of research and licensing activity of science and engineering faculty. Technological innovation: Generating economic results, Working Paper.

Trune, D.R., & Goslin, L.N. (1998). University technology transfer programs: A profit/loss analysis. *Technological Forecasting and Social Change, 57*(3), 197–204. http://dx.doi.org/10.1016/S0040-1625(97)00165-0

Walckiers, A. (2004). *Multidimensional screening and university output, part two: Should universities produce both research and teaching?* Mimeo.

Weiss, C.H. (1979). The many meanings of research utilization. *Public Administration Review, 39*(5), 426–31. http://dx.doi.org/10.2307/3109916

Wenger, E., McDermott, K., & Snyder, W. (2002). *Cultivating communities of practice*. Cambridge, MA: Harvard Business School Press.
Winter, G.W., & Szulanski, G. (2001). Replication as strategy. *Organization Science, 12*(6), 730–43. http://dx.doi.org/10.1287/orsc.12.6.730.10084
Yin, R., & Moore, G.B. (1988). Lessons on the utilization of research from nine case experiences in the natural hazards field, knowledge in society. *International Journal of Knowledge Transfer and Utilization, 1*(3), 25–44.
Zucker, L.G., Darby, M.R., & Armstrong, J. (2002). Commercializing knowledge: University science, knowledge capture, and firm performance in biotechnology. *Management Science, 48*(1), 138–53. http://dx.doi.org/10.1287/mnsc.48.1.138.14274

4 Evidence-Informed Public Policy Decision-Making

PETER C. COYTE

The CHSRF/CIHR Chair in Health Care Settings and Canadians was established in 2000 to build research capacity based on a priority triad of (1) focused research in applied health economics that pertains to health service finance, delivery, and organization across a range of settings; (2) innovative trainee education and mentorship in research and knowledge transfer; and (3) enhanced linkage and exchange with decision-makers. Research activities represent the coordinating hub for education and mentoring activities as well as for the linkage and exchange pursuits assembled under the auspices of the chair's program. In essence, the chair's program was designed, and has been periodically modified, to support knowledge capacity enhancement by: (1) generating new researchers who conduct more research; (2) enhancing the capacity of decision-makers to be effective participants in the knowledge production process; and (3) providing a forum for knowledge communication, dissemination, and uptake.

The chair's program has been built on a platform of interdisciplinary collaboration and thereby represents a departure from a more traditional single-discipline approach to health research training. It aims to bridge the knowledge and communication gaps that exist among researchers from various relevant disciplines and health professions as it prepares trainees who are able to understand and improve the new configurations of people, places, and technologies associated with healthcare in the twenty-first century. The demand from policy-makers, industry, and the public for enhanced research capacity in healthcare is immediate and critical. To meet it, program participants conduct exemplary research that contributes to the development and maintenance of humane, equitable, effective, and efficient healthcare for all Canadians.

In this chapter, I emphasize the chair's activities related to cultivation and advancement of evidence for policy decision-making and, more specifically, the role the chair's program played in knowledge dissemination and translation. My focus is on just one aspect of the role of evidence in influencing policy and practice, specifically, its role within law and Canadian jurisprudence. I discuss two exemplars. The first highlights the pedagogic role for evidence creation and dissemination within the chair's program. The second concerns an examination of evidence itself in immigration policy; specifically, what constitutes legitimate evidence and who has the authority, credibility, and expertise to present such evidence.

I illustrate non-traditional mechanisms for knowledge translation and describe the enhanced learning experience for trainees who actively participate in both knowledge creation and dissemination. I conclude with a range of important lessons for knowledge translation.

Evidence Creation and Translation

In this section, I discuss the contribution of the chair's program in its interactions with the law and Canadian jurisprudence within the context of knowledge production and transfer/translation among multiple networks, including trainees in the classroom, peer-reviewed journals, media, legal professionals, and the court. Specifically, I outline the process of knowledge creation and dissemination associated with my acquisition of evidence to guide legal and policy decision-making for provincial governments contemplating service expansion for children with autism. I conclude with a discussion of the outcomes for the trainees and the chair associated with this project.

From the Classroom to the Courtroom

Under the supervision of the chair and Dr Wendy Ungar, an associate professor and senior scientist at the Hospital for Sick Children in Toronto, and as part of a graduate course requirement during the fall of 2002, a team of three master's of science students evaluated the long-term cost-effectiveness of extending intensive behavioural intervention therapy to all children with autism in Ontario. At that time, the province provided funding for about one-third of autistic children, and there was substantial debate about the magnitude of its commitment to increase such funding and expand access to such services for children older than six years of age.

Given the paucity of effectiveness and costing data that pertain to the services offered to autistic children, the wide variations in public funding, and the associated uneven burden placed on families with autistic children, there was an urgent need for evidence to inform policy decision-making. As civil proceedings were in motion between families with autistic children and Ontario concerning the age limit on receiving provincial assistance, the research findings proved to be a useful contribution to that debate.

The trainees' scholarly analysis demonstrated that expanding therapy to all children with autism would result in potential cost savings of $172.5 million. At the conclusion of the graduate course, Dr Ungar and I worked tirelessly with the trainees to restructure the paper for scholarly submission (Motiwala, Gupta, Lilly, Ungar, & Coyte, 2006) and use by legal decision-makers representing both sides in the civil suit. By offering the report to the plaintiffs and to the government in April 2003, the trainees fulfilled the commitment to impartiality they had made at the outset of their work. Moreover, in order to accomplish the research training objectives that underlie the chair's program, trainees are offered assistance and supports to produce in situ evidence-based research, and are expected to champion the uptake of such findings by diverse legal, policy, and advocate stakeholders. Consequently, involvement of stakeholders in the research process and as audiences for the dissemination of findings such as those from the trainee's analysis is integral to the chair's program.

The research was admitted as evidence in *Wynberg v Ontario* on 17 September 2003 by lawyers for the plaintiffs, who alleged that the province was pursuing discriminatory treatment of children with autism. On the basis of my scholarly track record, I was called as an expert witness to testify to the veracity of the trainees' findings and support the legitimacy of the work. The trainees valued this level of mentorship; as one commented, "I guessed that if he was going to stand up in court and defend our project, then he must have thought it was really strong. I appreciated that" (Coyte, 2003).

After I appeared as a witness, without chattel, the Ontario Superior Court of Justice commissioned the research team, in January 2004, to reanalyse the cost-effectiveness of services to children with autism in light of new data disclosed by the Ontario Ministry of Community and Social Services. These data revealed higher treatment costs and fewer eligible children who would be served by an expanded program. Consequently, while the overall conclusions that service expansion saves costs were unchanged, the revised report demonstrated that the cost savings attributable to expansion were smaller, at $96.6 million, than the earlier figure of $172.5 million. The research team submitted this revised report to lawyers for the plaintiffs and the Ontario Superior Court announced its verdict on 1 April 2005. The court decided that Ontario had acted in a discriminatory manner by terminating funding when autistic children reached six years of age, and ordered the province to provide funding for older children.

This project demonstrates integrated research, education/mentorship, and linkage/exchange achievements. Through my (and Dr Ungar's) tutelage, trainees generated relevant and timely evidence that concerned the costs and consequences of health and social care for autistic children. This evidence had direct implications for decision-making and was promptly disseminated to and translated for a range of stakeholders. Dissemination was supported by involvement in the civil action, oral and poster presentations, and eventually in the preparation and publication of a manuscript.

Work for the trainees did not end with the decision by the Ontario Superior Court. In just over three years since the beginning of the graduate course, the trainees received advice on formatting the report in a style suitable for submission and consideration for publication in a peer-reviewed journal with an academic audience. The trainees were supported and assisted in responding to the evaluations of anonymous reviewers and editors as part of the peer-review process. Their findings were published in the January 2006 issue of *Healthcare Policy* (Motiwala et al., 2006). But matters did not end there.

In the meantime, the province of Ontario appealed the decision of the Ontario Superior Court, and the civil suit was under review by the Ontario Court of Appeal when the article was published in *Healthcare Policy*. As part of the case under appeal, I was charged with establishing the relationship between the findings in the original report that was subject of testimony in September 2003 and those in the article that appeared in *Healthcare Policy* in 2006. This resulted in the creation of a further affidavit and cross-examination in May 2006 that described the manner in which the advent of revised data from the Ministry of Community and Social Services changed the findings, and the review process changed the way they were reported. The concluding section of the affidavit indicates that, notwithstanding the modifications, the published article confirms the findings in the initial report.

Following this affidavit, the *Globe and Mail* ran an article on 6 June 2006 entitled, "Reopen autism case, Ontario asks court." The article indicated that the Ontario government was "seeking to reopen a major Court of Appeal case involving special treatment for autistic children, claiming that an expert witness [Dr Coyte] has undergone a dramatic change of heart about costs associated with treatment" (Mankin, 2006). The research team was not asked to comment on the story either prior or subsequent to its publication, and the newspaper did not publish the response by the research team that explained the changes were in part due to the provincial government's original non-disclosure of data. On 7 July 2006, the Ontario Court of Appeal ruled in favour of the province of Ontario.

Outcomes for the Trainees

Trainees learned first-hand the powerful influence that careful research-based economic evaluation can exert on legal outcomes and policy development. Mary Eberts, legal counsel for the plaintiffs, stated that the 2003 report is the "only Canadian cost-benefit analysis of any of the autism support services, and supports the conclusions of U.S. studies consulted during the early planning stages of the Ontario Intensive Early Intervention Program (IEIP). [The report] has contributed to keeping the IEIP on its initial trajectory, and even improving it."

Trainees also had the rare opportunity to participate in a project that exemplified the use of research evidence as a mechanism in the dialogue between courts and legislatures. A critical part of this dialogue involves the use of scientific evidence to facilitate the interaction between the court's role in interpreting the Charter of Rights and legislative goals as set out by democratically elected politicians. In other words, the trainees' 2003 report and 2006 article were key pieces of evidence that the court and the government used to reconcile "the individualistic values of the Charter with the accomplishment of social and economic policies enacted for the benefit of the community as a whole" (Hogg & Thornton, 1999, p. 22).

Finally, this experience gave the involved trainees critical, real-world experience in knowledge translation across disciplines. They had to respond to the genuine confusion evinced by the judicial system when faced with a paucity of knowledge concerning the cost and consequences of publicly funded services. This judicial learning helped them to understand the effects of scholarly dialogue and negotiation between authors and peer reviewers in the course of securing publication. Furthermore, the trainees acquired first-hand experience of the manner in which media sometimes distorts information, and how such actions may be used to influence judicial decisions.

Outcomes for the Chair

My experience of being called as an expert witness in this case also required me to begin to provide ongoing mentoring and support for the trainees' knowledge translation activities. When evidence-based research is translated into non-legal expert evidence through uptake by legal decision-makers, it is often the "credibility of the (expert) witness as a moral person" that is "crucial" to the law's acceptance of a study as credible (Valverde, 2007, p. 84). In this case, although the court was apprised that a graduate exercise in real-world economic evaluation was the genesis of the 2003 report, it was my qualification as an expert health economist that the court needed to accept the validity of the original, and subsequently revised but convergent, claims. Clearly, all current and future proponents of knowledge translation (particularly in the context of, but not limited to, Canadian jurisprudence) must recognize that the extent and depth of their moral standing is an important component in successfully engaging in real-world knowledge translation efforts.

Evidence that Informs and Evidence that Clouds Public Policy Decisions

Curiosity has traditionally driven the research process. While there is still ample scope for curiosity-driven research in the health research enterprise, the scales have shifted towards directed or goal-driven research (Gomory, 1994). Whether attributed to focused calls for research by granting agencies or to the increasingly common requirement that research be pursued in partnership with decision-maker organizations that are often directly involved in the process and funding, the dominant trend has been towards directed research. This trend has also resulted in a quantum shift towards the expectation that research findings will inform policy decision-making. While the study discussed in the previous section falls under the heading of curiosity-driven research, notwithstanding the interactions with decision-makers, in this section I address a study characterized as directed research. Then, I compare and contrast the experiences under each type of research regime for both the chair's program and the constituent components of evidence used for policy decision-making.

Immigration Applicants in Poor Health Need Not Apply

In this section, I describe a project funded by the Ontario HIV Treatment Network (OHTN) that sought to improve the transparency and quality of information used in the immigration adjudication process. The Canadian Immigration and Refugee Protection Act (IRPA) of 2001 (Department of Justice Canada, 2001) outlines the conditions under which individuals may be granted or denied admission to Canada. Section 38(1) of the IRPA stipulates that applications for residence may be rejected if an applicant's health "is likely" to be a danger to public health or public safety or if s/he "might reasonably be expected to cause excessive demand on Canadian health or social services." Subsection 1(1) of the Immigration and Refugee Protection Regulations defines "excessive demand":

> (a) a demand on health services or social services for which the anticipated costs would likely exceed average Canadian per capita health services and social services costs over a period of five consecutive years immediately following the most recent medical examination required by these Regulations, unless there is evidence that significant costs are likely to be incurred beyond that period, in which case the period is no more than 10 consecutive years; or
>
> (b) a demand on health services or social services that would add to existing waiting lists and would increase the rate of mortality and morbidity in Canada as a result of the denial or delay in the provision of those services to Canadian citizens or permanent residents. (Department of Justice Canada, 2002)

Notwithstanding the IRPA and its regulations, the criteria used by immigration officers in applying these provisions are unclear. Moreover, the quality and currency of the clinical, epidemiological, and economic evidence used to support immigration officers' decisions have never been comprehensively assessed. Consequently, there is tremendous room to contribute to the informed use of evidence in the immigration adjudication process in general, and for persons with specific illnesses and conditions in particular.

In January 2008, I, in concert with a range of community and legal stakeholders, initiated a project designed to assess Canadian immigration decisions and the evidence used to make a determination of medical inadmissibility due to excessive demand on Canadian health or social services. This research synthesis and knowledge dissemination project brought together a wide range of community activists interested in greater clarity and quality in the immigration adjudication process.

Ten trainees I supervised participated in this project, and thereby advanced the research training objectives of my program as chair. Eight of these trainees were high school students who had demonstrated significant academic promise and were enrolled in the University of Toronto's mentorship program, one was an accomplished second-year undergraduate student, and one was a talented doctoral candidate. Each pursued different aspects of the research. The undergraduate trainee interviewed stakeholders from the legal and policy communities regarding the processes used to make, challenge, and defend a determination of medical inadmissibility. She also conducted a structured review of the literature pertaining to medical inadmissibility. One high school trainee examined how the Community Reference Committee, composed of community activists, influenced the knowledge transfer process; three high school trainees reviewed the international literature on health-related barriers to international migration; three other high school trainees assessed the potential economic burden on Canadian health and social services associated with immigrants with hepatitis B or diabetes; and one high school trainee designed a mathematical model to assess the trajectory of healthcare costs for individuals with end-stage renal disease. The doctoral trainee developed methods to measure excessive demand using key concepts from Canadian jurisprudence, statistics, and economics, and applied such methods to markers of disease progression for persons with HIV that would warrant a determination of medical inadmissibility on the basis of excessive demand.

I acquired overall funding for this research through a special request for board-directed funds from the OHTN, an advocacy network composed of community groups, health professionals, persons with HIV, researchers, and activists. It is independent of government but receives funding from the Ontario Ministry of Health and Long-Term

Care. In reviewing my application, the board established a range of funding conditions that the project needed to satisfy. As key requirements, community groups had to participate on the research team and the Community Reference Committee (CRC) had to be involved in knowledge translation. While funding was welcome, the advocacy groups' involvement in the research and dissemination processes raised a range of potential concerns. Indeed, though the project began as primarily curiosity-driven, it evolved to one share many characteristics commonly found in directed research.

One of the key characteristics of curiosity-driven research is the latitude afforded to the principal investigator(s) in terms of hiring personnel, establishing work plans consistent with the study objectives, selecting methods of inquiry, interpreting study findings, developing dissemination strategies (including the target audiences), and curating findings to privilege in the dissemination process. Probably because the stakes were high for all participants through inquiry into the immigration adjudication process, and specifically into medical inadmissibility for groups with specific medical conditions, membership in the research team as well as in the management of the project evolved between my original submission and the OHTN's funding announcement. In the end, two co-principal investigators managed the project, the research team included community activists, and a CRC was established to provide advice on study design, data collection, the interpretation of findings, and dissemination.

Research that examines the immigration adjudication process may result in both controversial and sensitive findings – not only for immigration applicants and their Canadian sponsors, but also for other communities. For example, quantifying and casually disseminating the health or social care costs of persons with HIV may cause any government to develop even more restrictive immigration policies or may cause increased stigma and discrimination against people with HIV. While it is impossible to prevent all negative outcomes, our harm reduction activities included the establishment of the CRC and involvement of community activists on the research team. Preparedness planning for the most vulnerable and affected groups was based on the prerelease of potentially damaging information before any possible public backlash.

Ultimately, the shift from a primarily curiosity-driven research project to a more directed one did not have a measurable effect on either the research training or the research production objectives of the chair's program. The trainees were intimately involved with the research and were full members of the team. Their activities were not subject to scrutiny by the whole research team, as the chair formed a buffer between the trainees and both advocacy members of the research team and the CRC. In addition, as the study's findings were consistent with the objectives of the advocacy groups involved, those groups did not ask either the research team as a whole, or individual researchers in particular, to revisit the findings. Moreover, were the findings to be disputed, mechanisms had been developed to (1) review, and possibly modify, the study findings if there was compelling evidence to support revision; and (2) include harm reduction measures in the dissemination strategy.

I did not decide to act as a buffer between trainees and advocacy groups lightly, as it did limit the trainees' learning opportunities and professional growth. I made the decision for three reasons: first, to streamline communication channels and ensure that participants were informed of the research as well as the checks and balances used when undertaking research; second, to preserve the trainees' time, as interactions with advocacy groups were time-intensive; and finally, to balance the potential learning opportunities for the trainees (through their interaction with advocacy groups) with the potential for contamination of the research process. Obviously, these decisions were specific to time and place, and were enormously dependent on the knowledge and understanding of the concerned people and communities. As this was my first major involvement with such advocacy groups as chair, I erred on the side of caution. If I were to repeat a similar exercise, I would contemplate more interactions and exchanges.

Important Knowledge Translation Lessons

The chair's program provides a focused research project as a platform to advance education and mentoring goals for trainees and foster linkage and exchange with policy decision-makers. These integrated, collaborative, and interdisciplinary activities form the hallmark of the chair's research training program. While the autism and immigration projects show the variety of research projects pursued, they are also important examples of integration and knowledge exchange. Both research projects made significant contributions to public policy decision-making, and together they indicate six important knowledge translation lessons (discussed in part by Lilly & Coyte, 2007).

Lesson One: Research Teams Must Be Responsive to Evolving Public Priorities

In the autism project, less than one year transpired between recognizing the research opportunity and submitting the final report. This rapid response offered insufficient time to pursue or receive research grants, and also required students to realign their research priorities for the duration of the project. The immigration project also had less than twelve months between the submission for funding and the project's completion. This quick turnaround was partly due to incentives and the pressing need for evidence to inform policy, the law, and Canadian jurisprudence. In both instances, the chair enabled me to take the time necessary to mentor students through each project. Each project was embedded in a specific context, and so their results may not apply to other contexts. Nevertheless, it is important to consider and foster ways the research community may improve its responsiveness while maintaining scientific integrity.

Lesson Two: Opportunities to Effect Public Policy Decision-Making Exist

Involvement in health and, more generally, public policy decision-making takes considerable initiative on the part of researchers and is frequently pursued without reward, financial or otherwise. At times, researchers may feel that the academic processes and markers of success, such as conference presentations and peer-reviewed publications, are sufficient knowledge translation strategies. However, experience with the two projects described in this chapter suggests that such academic achievements are often far removed from courtroom testimony or immigration adjudication. It is doubtful whether the two worlds would have met had a researcher not taken the lead in the autism case and had the OHTN board not funded the immigration project. Moreover, in effecting change, the academic process seems easier to manage and offers fewer uncertainties than either legal proceedings or modifying public policies and regulations.

Lesson Three: Knowledge Translation Strategies Should Be Multilayered and Concurrent

Prior to pursuing scholarly publication, the research teams made tailored reports to stakeholders, entered evidence as testimony, and gave presentations to academic and stakeholder communities. In the case of the autism project, scientific publication was the final knowledge translation strategy to be realized, and the article became publicly available only after the Ontario Superior Court of Justice delivered its ruling. The immigration project followed a similar process of knowledge translation. Moreover, while that project was equally contentious and had a similar potential for harm, the research team pursued deliberate preparedness planning and harm reduction in designing the dissemination strategy.

Lesson Four: Knowledge Translation Activities Should Begin at a Project's Inception (or Sooner)

To maximize the impact and relevance of research findings, it is crucial to initiate knowledge translation as soon as possible. The initial drive for the autism project came from a parent with an autistic child and was clearly relevant to lawyers representing both the provincial government and parents. The study was strengthened by its independence and its opportunity to consider various perspectives throughout the data analysis period. In the case of the immigration project, legal counsel for individuals deemed medically inadmissible for immigration championed the study, and the findings spread within that community. While decision-makers from Citizenship and Immigration Canada were also invited to participate, they declined formal involvement. However, officials at Citizenship and Immigration Canada were apprised of the research activities, tentative research results, and findings.

Lesson Five: Knowledge Translation Should Be Fully Integrated into the Graduate Curricula

At the time the trainees pursued work on the projects described in this chapter, particularly that on autism, knowledge translation as a formal discipline was relatively unknown – there were no graduate (or undergraduate) level courses and few training opportunities. Five of the seven trainees who participated in either project had limited experience working with stakeholders and decision-makers as they were high school students, undergraduates, or enrolled in a master's of science program. These projects were exemplars of "trial by fire" for all trainees, but particularly for those with limited exposure to the field of knowledge translation. Fortunately, there have been significant revisions to the curricula. Several institutions now offer knowledge translation courses that expose students to both conceptual and applied knowledge translation, and more students have the option to take a practicum. In particular, an integral component of the chair's program is participation in a knowledge translation course that pertains to the financing, delivery, and organization of home- and community-based healthcare. Trainees select policy- and program-relevant research and translate it into an accessible format for decision-makers. They provide synopses in two formats: headlines and conclusions crystallize the take-home messages of the research in a few sentences, while thumbnail summaries condense the background, methods, findings, and conclusions of the research into quick-to-use, single-page overviews that include reference information. In doing so, they learn the basics of knowledge translation. Notwithstanding these changes, knowledge translation remains a relatively marginal component of many students' training experience.

Lesson Six: Knowledge Translation in Legal Environments Requires Additional Skills

Not unlike the peer-review process, research results that become legal evidence are subject to intense scrutiny, and sources of potential bias are heavily investigated. However, unlike the scientific process, the legal environment also holds witnesses accountable for any possible perception of bias, even if it does not exist. Because the research team's involvement in both the autism and immigration projects originated from meetings with an interested party, team members were very sensitive to these issues. Participants were careful to operate in an open, transparent, and neutral manner; to use data available to all parties; and to provide all parties with identical information simultaneously. Finally, testifying as an expert witness (in the case of the autism project) can be quite unlike any other professional experiences of academic life. I recommend that researchers called as expert witnesses seek orientation about what to expect, perhaps in a vein similar to media training.

Conclusion

The chair's program has used research projects as the integrating mechanism to advance education and mentoring goals and foster linkage and exchange with policy decision-makers. While research may be narrowly viewed as an inquiry that generates evidence, the chair's program has adopted a broader interpretation of research as a platform for education and mentoring as well as a forum for knowledge exchange.

To enhance knowledge uptake, it is crucial to involve decision-makers at the outset of the research process, and especially in the articulation of the questions to be addressed. Moreover, immersing trainees in a process of knowledge generation that involves decision-makers and has the potential for immediate uptake yields excitement, caution, and industry, and helps to develop a new form of researcher: one that savours the involvement of decision-makers and is stimulated by the potential for knowledge uptake. The chair's program reflects this paradigm shift in knowledge production and distribution. Trainees are no longer merely inputs into the research production process. By constructing – and in the process socializing – a new type of researcher, and by enhancing the capacity of decision-makers to be both effective participants in the research process and users of evidence, the chair's program emphasizes knowledge capacity enhancement.

REFERENCES

Coyte, P.C. (2003). *2003 CHSRF/CIHR Health Services Chair report.* Unpublished document.

Department of Justice Canada. (2001). *Immigration and refugee protection act of 2001.* Retrieved 28 July 2009 from http://laws-lois.justice.gc.ca/eng/acts/I-2.5/index.html

Department of Justice Canada. (2002). *Immigration and refugee protection regulations.* Retrieved 28 July 2009 from http://laws-lois.justice.gc.ca/eng/regulations/SOR-2002-227/FullText.html

Gomory, R.E. (1994). The US government's role in science and technology. *Research Management Review, 7*(1), 1–13.

Hogg, P.W., & Thornton, A.A. (1999). The charter dialogue between courts and legislatures. *Policy Options,* (April 1999), 19–22.

Lilly, M.B., & Coyte, P.C. (2007). *"When research evidence becomes legal evidence: Knowledge translation in the courtroom." Submitted to CIHR Institute of Neurosciences, Mental Health and Addictions (INMHA).* KT Casebook.

Mankin, K. (2006, June 6). Reopen autism case, Ontario asks court. *Globe and Mail.*

Motiwala, S.S., Gupta, S., Lilly, M.B., Ungar, W.J., & Coyte, P.C. (2006). The cost-effectiveness of expanding intensive behavioural intervention to all autistic children in Ontario. *Health Policy (Amsterdam)*, *1*(2), 135–51. Medline:19305662

Valverde, M. (2007). Theoretical and methodological issues in the study of legal knowledge practices. In A. Sarat, L. Douglas, & M.M. Umphrey (Eds.), *How law knows* (pp. 72–92). Standford, CA: Stanford University Press.

5 The Mediating Role of Research in Shaping the Socio-Health Space

LOUISE POTVIN

In Canada, there is an increasing awareness that interventions that aim to improve population health should be studied and evaluated using scientific methods (Potvin, Hawe, & Di Ruggiero, 2009). The knowledge produced by such population health intervention research is critical for orienting action and informing policy decisions (Butler-Jones, 2009). However, such research also has a less known and discussed potential application, which I discuss in this chapter. The participatory evaluation research program implemented under the umbrella of my CHSRF/CIHR Chair in Community Approaches and Health Inequalities illustrates how population health intervention research can mediate collaborations between organizations with different mandates and resources. More specifically, when state agencies such as public health organizations develop collaborative programs with community organizations to plan and implement interventions that address social determinants of health, the presence of a third party, in the form of a participatory research team, modifies the relationships between the partners. In this chapter, I reflect on the conditions that made it possible for the chair to play an active role in the construction of the socio-health space.

The chair's main decision-making partner is the director of public health for the Greater Montreal Area, whose organization comprises more than 200 public health professionals. In 1998, in his first annual report on the health of Montrealers, the director produced critical data on variations in health indicators across Montreal boroughs that showed, for example, an eleven-year discrepancy in life expectancy between the most and least affluent neighbourhoods (Direction de la santé publique de Montréal, 1998). Ten years before Canada's chief public health officer did so (Chief Public Health Officer, 2008), this report acknowledged the influence of social conditions on population health and identified the reduction of social health inequalities as a top priority. One of the main strategies developed in response to this priority was through various partnership programs with regional key actors such as the City of Montreal, United Way of Montreal, and other ministries' regional directorates to support local development projects by local coalitions that rely heavily on the leadership and participation of community organizations.

The public health innovative practices that support this strategy suggest that professionals work closely with local community organizations to pursue goals that may not be immediately associated with health. When I developed the chair's program with the Montreal director of public health, we decided that the research part of the program would investigate the innovative practices and programs that contribute to the general public health strategy to reduce social health inequalities (Potvin, Lessard, & Fournier, 2002). To achieve this goal, we developed a multidisciplinary research team that collaborated with community organizations and with researchers and practitioners from the Montreal Public Health Department. In this chapter I show how, and under which conditions, this participatory research program mediated the elaboration of the socio-health space (Fassin, 1998).

The New Public Health, the Local Scene, and the Socio-Health Space

The Ottawa Charter (WHO, 1986) proposes a new agenda for public health intervention, an agenda that has been labelled the "New Public Health" (Ashton & Seymour, 1988). In addition to defining five strategies of action, the charter offers three ideas that led to the "third revolution of public health" (Breslow, 1999, p. 1,031; Potvin & McQueen, 2007). First, it explicitly states that health is created in everyday life and out of local conditions. The charter identifies peace, shelter, food, and income, among other factors, as prerequisites for health, and indicates that specific social conditions, now recognized as the social determinants of health (WHO Commission on Social Determinants of Health, 2008), are associated with improved population health. Second, it identifies a core set of humanist principles and values such as equity, empowerment, and participation as necessary underlying processes for health promotion (Potvin, McQueen, & Hall, 2008). Finally, it calls for intersectoral action. Health promotion interventions aim to improve social conditions, and so they should be developed by large and inclusive coalitions with the capacity to reach out well beyond the health sector and transform local conditions in order to improve the health of all groups in a population (Potvin, Gendron, Bilodeau, & Chabot, 2005).

Twenty years after the Ottawa Charter, and recognizing the complexity of the task of promoting health as a resource for daily life, the Bangkok Charter for Health Promotion in a Globalised World (WHO, 2005) stated that public health needs to form alliances with both private enterprises and also community organizations as two networks with which public health needs to develop alliances in order to promote population health (Kickbusch, 2002). Such multi-network alliances, especially those involving community organizations, are increasingly promoted as a means for public health interventions to reach vulnerable populations or to address health inequalities (Frohlich & Potvin, 2008). Indeed, public health organizations increasingly perceive community organizations, often created in response to the social needs of the most vulnerable groups, as the point of entry to access and serve marginalized populations who traditionally experience difficulties in their interactions with institutions. Thus, public health organizations more often partner with other local agencies and design various incentives for community organizations to broaden their mandates to include health and related resources and services.

As a reflection on those local partnerships that foster conditions that promote health, Didier Fassin (1998) suggests that on the local scene, health provides meaning to action and interactions. Health is no longer exclusive to the health sector; it is a shared responsibility, not only for a number of state activities, such as education, transportation, social development, family affairs, justice, and others, but also for community organizations and private corporations. For example, commentators suggest that in Western societies, non-medical health products, such as healthy food, magazines, and body-care services, represent a market of several hundred billion dollars annually (Kickbusch, 2009). As for community organizations, their endemic lack of sustainable funding often leads them to bid for health sector funding programs to partner in developing targeted health programs and services.

The Montreal Public Health Department is engaged in two types of partnerships. One type involves other governmental agencies from non-health sectors, such as education, transportation, or employment, which provide services and programs that affect social determinants of health. I label these partnerships intersectoral action because they are formed with representatives from different areas of public administration. Such partnerships are created to overcome the limitations of specialized actions constrained by borders that define the stakes and expertise associated with specific public sectors (Bilodeau, 2005). Administrative structures and processes that allow the parties involved to cross those borders and share resources and expertise characterize them. In Quebec, for example, regional administrative commissions have mandates to coordinate the regional action of various government ministries and agencies in order to promote an integrated and coherent vision of economic and/or social development (Gouvernement du Québec, 2009).

The second type of partnership involves members who belong to organizations with different operating modes. There are three broad categories of organizations that operate in the public space (Godbout, 2005). First, private organizations produce goods and services that are accessible through economic transactions that cover both the production costs and profit margin. Such organizations are accountable to shareholders, and their value and that of the goods they produce is subject to market fluctuations. Second, state agencies and institutions provide services and programs that are accessible according to an explicit set of rigid rules, with or without a nominal fee that may or may not cover the cost of production. Such organizations are accountable to an elected body, either directly or indirectly via a board of directors. Usually in liberal economies, state agencies provide either universal services that are deemed necessary to ensure the well-being of the entire population, such as infant vaccination, or specialized services to well-defined targeted populations that cannot access certain services through the market, such as social housing. Third, the alternatively labelled community, not-for-profit, or non-governmental organization provides goods, services, and programs through membership and co-optation. Groups of individuals found these organizations to pursue interests specific to themselves and their volunteers. Such organizations are accountable to their members and build valuable social connections through the goods and services they provide (Godbout, 2000). For example, housing associations and cooperatives provide goods (in this case, housing) that derive value both from the market price and also from the social connectedness associated with the arrangement. Multi-network coalitions are collaborative partnerships that draw members from at least two different categories of organizations.

This distinction between intersectoral and multi-network coalitions is useful because the politics involved in the latter are usually much more complex than those involved in the former. Intersectoral collaborations involve separate agencies that all operate within the same bureaucratic structure, and so they require bureaucratic agreements that define mandates, structures, and processes. Although issues like areas of jurisdiction, resource imbalance, or differing organizational cultures may emerge from time to time and slow down the work of such coalitions, they are ultimately driven by political decisions made outside of their bureaucratic operational space, which facilitates the negotiation of modus operandi that satisfy participating agencies (Berkeley & Springett, 2006a). For example, the leaders of Montreal regional offices of several Quebec ministries (such as health and social welfare, education, sports and leisure, municipal affairs, and employment), negotiated a collaborative agreement with the City of Montreal to develop and coordinate social development projects in a local low-income neighbourhood. Following this agreement, the role of the steering committee, made of local partners and responsible for the implementation of the project, was essentially technical. The committee had to operate within the agreement and budget that had been negotiated at the political level (Borvil & Kishchuk, 2007).

Multi-network partnerships, for their part, usually operate in more conflicting spaces, mainly as a result of the divergent operating logics between categories of organizations, and of the power imbalance that often characterizes partnership projects between state agencies and community organizations (Nelisse, 1994). Indeed, state agencies often approach multi-network collaborations with both an agenda to orient the action and the resources to implement it. The agenda derives its strength and legitimacy from the expert knowledge it is based on and from the agency's legal mandate. Resources are usually made available commensurate to the project's priority within the agency. Except for periodic evaluations and audits, state agencies have recurrent yearly budgets that are fairly stable and allow them to plan their operation and development. Community organizations, however, are plagued with an endemic lack of resources, and although their membership base provides them with strong internal legitimacy, their capacity to reach out other groups in the population is often limited due to limited resources (Berkeley & Springett, 2006a).

Alliances between public health and community organizations constitute a novelty for health practitioners. There is no written manual for these partnerships. They often face the romantic conception that good will and positive attitude is sufficient to smooth conflicts and guarantee success (Boutiller, Cleverly, & Labonte, 2000). The partnerships are often defined by the institutional actor and are vertical: the role of the community partners is often seen as mostly instrumental to the pursuit of health objectives, independent of their own objectives. Community organizations often cruelly lack the financial resources and technical expertise that institutional actors bring to the partnership, which confers to the latter structural power over the former, even if institutional practitioners often prefer to act as if such power imbalance does not exist or is irrelevant in the pursuit of the shared objectives. On the other side of the equation, community organizations often function more horizontally and are closer and more responsive to members' interests and needs. They often see the alignment of their goals to those of partner state agencies – necessary to access funding and expertise – as a betrayal of their original mandate that is justifiable only as a survival strategy. They are often blind to the assets they bring to the partnership as a legitimacy guarantee and a mandatory pathway through which state agencies access vulnerable populations.

Thus, the constitution of the socio-health space, a space of collaboration and innovation for the new public health, appears hazardous and criss-crossed by diverging interests. The capacity for public institutions, such as public health, to mobilize the civil society in their effort to improve population health is much more limited than what transpires from the literature. In their study of local implementation strategies of national programs, MacKian, Elliott, Busby, and Popay (2003) show that the vertical logic of state programs gets lost in the fuzzier and less orderly world of local dynamics. State agencies cannot program the local reality at will, even if they have the best of intentions and doing so will benefit local people. It is highly frustrating for decision-makers to enter partnerships in which their expertise and resources are contested. Conversely, local community organizations cannot use the resources that come with those partnerships and simply continue to pursue their own agendas. Accountability and evaluation mechanisms force them to operate within a logic that is not entirely compatible with their action-oriented and experience-informed modus operandi. Community organization staff often fail to see the relevance of evaluation and monitoring, which they perceive as controlling bureaucratic devices and obstacles to action and solutions (Laperrière & Zúñiga, 2006). Over and above their power differentials, there exist real cultural barriers to collaboration between community organizations and public health institutions (Berkeley & Springett, 2006a). In many instances partnerships fail, either because the creative tension generated by frustrated mutual expectations cannot be expressed – with the result that community organizations are instruments through which state agencies programs are delivered, unchanged, at a lower cost – or because those tensions evolve into full-fledged conflicts that lead to program implementation failure (Berkeley & Springett, 2006b).

Developing Socio-Health Spaces in Montreal Boroughs

The Quebec health reform of 1992 implemented the health sector decentralization agenda. This reform had major impacts on the organization of public health services. The public health responsibility was displaced from the thirty-two existing hospital-based departments of community health and transferred to eighteen newly created administrative health regions. In each region, under the leadership of a director of public health (the equivalent of a medical officer of health), a public health department was responsible for identifying public health priorities and developing and implementing programs in line with them. In the Montreal area, the director of public health became responsible for the health of the population of the whole Island of Montreal, a region that includes the downtown core and most suburbs. In 1998, the director's first report on the health of Montrealers was devoted to health inequalities, framing the reduction of health inequalities as the highest public health priority (Direction de la santé publique de Montréal, 1998; 2001). "My patient is the population of Montreal," the director of public health used to say, "and my patient is sick because poorer and less educated people cannot enjoy the same health as average Montrealers. Like any doctor would do, I have to pay attention to what makes my patient sick and try to get rid of it. Therefore poverty is a public health concern." In order to act on this priority, the director developed a series of programs with municipal and regional partners, making a point to become a relevant actor in various regional decision-making and policy orientation bodies, and to participate in various regional anti-poverty initiatives.

In agreement with this strategic direction, the Montreal Public Health Department joined United Way of Montreal and the City of Montreal to support the funding of local coalition tables in each of the Montreal boroughs. These coalitions were local networks of partners whose mandate was to establish consultation and dialogue mechanisms to develop action plans on local social and economic development issues. At that time, this program institutionalized the merging of two different funding mechanisms that operated on very different premises (Bujold, 2001).

One funding mechanism, under the joint responsibility of the Public Health Directorate and the City of Montreal, was the Healthy City Program. In agreement with WHO guidelines, this program funded local coalitions that included representatives from local community primary care organizations, other local institutions, and other community organizations. With agendas openly geared towards health objectives, those coalitions collaborated with government organizations at the local and regional levels. The second funding mechanism was the result of a joint program of the social development branch of the City of Montreal and United Way of Montreal. This program aimed to support local dialogue and communication between various community organizations that operated in socio-economically deprived local neighbourhoods. Montreal has a long history of community mobilization around community organizations that provide specialized and innovative support for action to various groups in situations of vulnerability, and at the same time pursue political agendas of citizen awareness-raising that often lead to tension with institutions. Structurally, such coalitions did not directly include representatives from local institutions such as municipal representatives or government agencies. The umbrella program is now called the Montreal Initiative to Support Local Development.

As a government agency, the Montreal Public Health Department gave the local development program a stronger preoccupation with accountability and evaluation. There was a need to demonstrate the results of public health investments. Early in the program, the department commissioned a researcher with the mandate of enrolling the local coalition tables into an evaluation research project. Despite the open intention to create a participatory space for this project, the local coalition tables' coordination committee rejected the project on the basis that the funding agencies determined the research questions and that there were no opportunities to question and examine the funding practices governing the program. The committee perceived evaluation as yet another control mechanism through which funding agencies could regulate and dominate the action of community organizations.

In 1999, when I began to develop my chair application in partnership with Montreal's director of public health, the director insisted that the chair program evaluate the local coalition tables. A core goal of the chair's research program is thus to study and produce knowledge from the Montreal Initiative to Support Local Development and to learn from those who operate the program locally.

Thus, from the beginning, the chair has operated a research program at the partnering interface of health and other sector institutions, local community organizations, and one charity. Each of these organizations pursues its own objectives as identified in its mandate, but all also agree that the initiative was a way to achieve such mandates – including those that address the social determinants of health. Additionally, controversies marked the relationships between some community organizations and the public health department. These controversies were the result of a history of difficult and tense relationships, but were also inherently associated with the power imbalance between public and community organizations and their different, if not divergent, modes of operation (Laforest & Phillips, 2001).

Controversy, Innovation, and Conflicting Collaboration

The appealing rhetoric of the Ottawa and Bangkok charters fails to recognize tensions and controversies associated with forming and mobilizing a network of organizations with varied perspectives in order to create local health promotion processes (Potvin, 2007). The sociology of translation examines how socio-technical networks composed of previously disparate entities are assembled and mobilized, and how the controversies and mediations that are part of such activities are also requirements for the development of social innovations (Akrich, Callon, & Latour 1988a; 1988b). The Actor Network Theory proposes a theoretical lens with which to understand how connections form and operate between previously unrelated entities in order to construct a social reality that will give them a new identity (Latour, 2005).

The mere coexistence of two entities within the same context does not ensure a connection. Callon (1986) argued that translation is necessary to connect previously unrelated and estranged entities. Translation is the process by which the identities, interests, and roles of previously unrelated elements are negotiated and aligned with one another to form a new socio-technical network. The actions of the chair and its research program facilitated translations between partners in order to create the socio-health space.

Indeed, research has shown that the local coalition tables that compose the program are quite heterogeneous (Sénécal, Herjean, & Cloutier, 2006). Those who originally belonged to the Healthy City program were more likely to be broader and to include representatives from public organizations and institutions such as community police, schools, local health centres, and social services, whereas those who originated from Montreal's social development program were usually exclusively composed of representatives from community organizations and citizens. The latter were more likely to have opposed the public health department's original evaluation attempts before the implementation of the chair program. They perceived that the capacity for coalitions that excluded representatives from state agencies to still receive funding through the program was at stake with the evaluation, while the public health department was perceived as promoting the Healthy City model for the tables – a model that is more inclusive of all neighbourhood organizations.

The space in which the chair's research program developed was thus populated by state agencies and community organizations, each trying to work out the best possible outcomes from a partnership characterized by tensions and controversies over acceptable networking (though they agreed that various coalition arrangements could be part of the program), evaluation, and monitoring mechanisms. Although the program's goals and objectives were clearly stated, there were difficulties in aligning the interests of the various parties involved, in part because state agencies and community organizations had inherently different operating modes. It was clear from the beginning of the chair that it had to acquire legitimacy as a scientific knowledge structure in a politicized space with a history of tension. Interestingly, the mechanisms that were implemented to enhance the chair's legitimacy and capacity to fulfil its mandate of conducting scientific research were also instrumental in aligning the interests of parties involved in the program.

According to the Actor Network Theory, uncertainties, controversies, and innovations are inherently linked to the expansion and consolidation of socio-technical networks (Callon, Lascoume, & Barthe, 2001). Consolidated networks are the result of multiple translations that establish roles and identities and stabilize connections. A stabilized network and its elements can be mobilized for coordinated action. Processes become routines and the various elements in the network work as intermediaries, in the sense that they carry on the action in a predictable way (Latour, 2005). In emerging and less stable networks, however, identities and roles between previously unconnected entities must be negotiated, and behaviours and actions of any entity with undetermined connections are less predictable as a result (Latour, 2005). In addition, the more distant and different the entities to be connected are at the beginning of the translation process, the more unstable and uncertain the network and, consequently, the more intensive the translation process required to mobilize the network into coordinated actions. In emerging networks, entities are mediators who act on the information and action to better match it with their interests (Latour, 2005).

The constitution of the socio-health space in which public health agencies develop processes and mechanisms to align their mandates with those of community organizations starts as an emerging network. There is no a priori reason for community organizations to spontaneously embrace the objectives pursued by public health. Community organizations have their own mandates developed in relationship with their membership, and any transformation of those mandates should require membership realignment. Indeed, when public health agencies offer program moneys to community organizations in order to carry out public health-related actions, what they do, in fact, is introduce into stabilized networks several new entities in the form of public health money, knowledge, values, and objectives with which entirely new connections need to be operated through series of translations in order to stabilize and transform the community organization's socio-technical network. This destabilization creates uncertainty and controversies within community organizations and among the new network they join. Until the network stabilizes, these organizations act as mediators; they do not necessarily behave in a way that the logic model of the program anticipated. This relationship between public agencies and community organizations is characterized by "conflicting cooperation" (Mantoura, Gendron, & Potvin, 2007). The relationship is cooperative because the parties involved know they must collaborate and develop shared interests in order to pursue their own mandates. At the same time, the relationship is conflicted because of the structural power imbalance between community organizations and state agencies, and also because the former are much more vulnerable and less stable than the latter.

The Mediating Role of the Chair in the Socio-Health Space

The chair is a research infrastructure composed of a chair holder (me), research collaborators, graduate students, and research coordinators. As an entity trying to connect with organizations in the socio-health space, we had to develop mechanisms to align the interests of researchers with those of practitioners in charge of interventions that address the social determinants of public health. We used three methods to help facilitate this translation process.

First, we created a research coordinator position with a job description very much like that of a translator. Day to day, this person facilitates information exchange between partnering community organizations, partnering state agencies, and researchers and graduate students from a variety of disciplines who are interested in conducting research in the socio-health space. From the sociology of translation guiding the practical development of this position, we learned that controversies can be managed only by considering diverse perspectives and types of knowledge (Callon, Lascoume, & Barthe, 2001). We found that the chair was an ideal structure to intensify exchanges in the socio-health space. First, as a research organization, the chair was credible and legitimate in its dealings with knowledge. Second, because the chair's main interest in the socio-health space was related not to orienting action but to producing knowledge about the conditions for developing action, the other parties perceived it not as a neutral entity but as a party whose main strategic arena was situated out of the socio-health space, in academia and scientific knowledge diffusion. In fact, the chair's main goal with regards to the Montreal Initiative to Support Local Development was its continuation in any form or direction, in order to be able to continue the study.

One of the chair's roles in the transformation of the socio-health space was to facilitate communications, to introduce and value assorted knowledge relevant to the various dimensions of the controversies, and to make sure that all parties could access all this knowledge. This translation function was key to the chair's work and took various forms. For example, all communication devices and knowledge and exchange events created and facilitated by the chair had to make room for knowledge and viewpoints that were representative of research, community partners, and state agency partners. This was true for the chair's advisory board, bulletin, and public seminar series. So, in the chair's program, knowledge exchange and translation is necessarily a multidirectional process in which a conversation developed with partners from three types of organizations.

Second, we developed a framework for research partnership agreements that was the product of an intense negotiation between spokespersons from state agencies, community organizations, and the chair (Bernier, Rock, Roy, Bujold, & Potvin, 2006). This agreement was instrumental in defining the roles and responsibilities of all parties involved in the chair's research (CACIS, 2002). Interestingly, as this work has shown, the social space of research is closely related to the social space of interventions. The history of relationships that develop in one space impacts those in the other (Mantoura, Gendron, & Potvin, 2007). This mechanism facilitates the development of reflexivity in all parties involved.

Reflexivity characterizes a subjective action that attempts to position itself in its context through translating and adapting its goals and with the constraints and possibilities of the environment in which it takes place. A reflexive action constantly moves, so the actors become aware of their position in time and space such that totally subjective or totally external points of view do not exist. Because our framework provides a reference for defining roles and responsibilities of various actors while, at the same time, it offers opportunities for new information to circulate more freely, our research program was instrumental in enhancing the reflexivity of all actors, including researchers, in the socio-health space (Hordijk & Baud, 2006). Our work shows that such a reflexive posture in participatory research has great potential to create conditions that facilitate the mutual trust, transparency, and communication necessary for the development of innovations (Mantoura, Gendron, & Potvin, 2007). Thus, researchers become mediators in the process of collective action, and participatory research can provide conditions that enhance the actors' potential for reflexive practices, making research a key stakeholder in the socio-health space.

Third, we implemented operational mechanisms to equalize the power relations in the research space, which had repercussions in the socio-health space. Although the chair's institutional partner was a public health organization, partners made it clear that the chair's research program would not be driven by the needs of this sole organization. Furthermore, we recognized that state agencies and public organizations have a longer tradition of interaction with research and were therefore more susceptible to adopt powerful positions and postures in the development of research projects. One of the first things the chair did was hold a series of face-to-face meetings with various potential research partners to establish that there was no preset research question. Meeting parties individually helped to establish connections and clarify the roles of all parties in the program's development. We also established that the participation of representatives from community organizations in all research activities would be reimbursed directly to the participating organizations at a level commensurate to

Figure 5.1 The Socio-Health Space

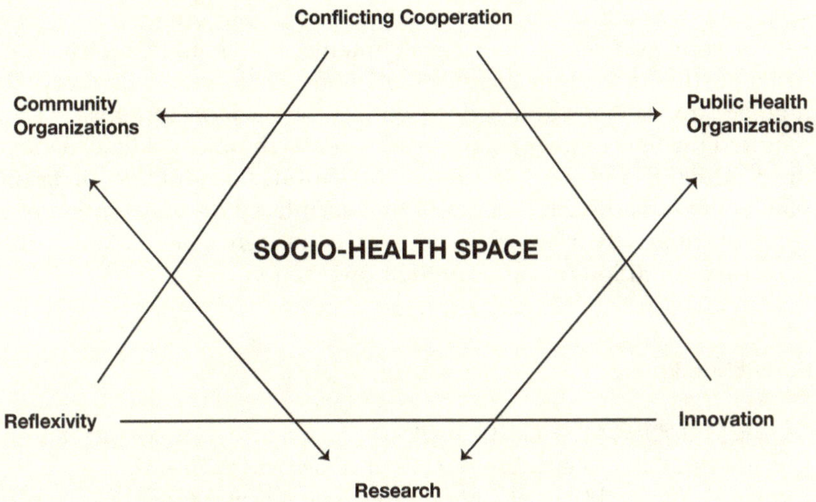

the average salary of professionals in such organizations. Professionals' job descriptions in most state agencies include some provision for participation in evaluation and research, and so we did not extend this practice to them.

Conclusion

The chair's research program has demonstrated that the socio-health space can be conceptualized as a socio-technical network. It is an assemblage of heteroclite entities that must be actively connected and aligned. These connections require negotiations and tradeoffs to become strong and stable. In the case of the socio-health space where public health organizations attempt to partner with community organizations, the power and resource imbalance results in multiple tensions that threaten the functioning of these already fragile alliances. The chair's program has shown how a research organization can facilitate the translation process necessary to support these new networks.

Figure 5.1 provides a model of the constitution of the socio-health space. In this space, research plays a key mediating role that allows the controversies inherent to the conflicting cooperation relationship between involved partners to be openly debated and critically appraised using all forms of knowledge available. Aware of the key role of controversies in new developments, the chair, as a structure, fostered the development of innovations that were necessary to regulate transactions and actions within the socio-health space. This required the development of innovative research practices that enabled the production and confrontation of the various forms of knowledge at play in the socio-health space, and thus facilitated the constitution of a space of reflexivity in which various partners were able to identify the necessary conditions to produce their own action.

REFERENCES

Akrich, M., Callon, M., & Latour, B. (1988a). A quoi tient le success des innovations? 1: L'art de l'intéressement. *Gérer et comprendre, 11,* 4–17.

Akrich, M., Callon, M., & Latour, B. (1988b). A quoi tient le success des innovations? 2: Le choix des porte-parole. *Annales de mines, 12,* 14–29.

Ashton, J., & Seymour, H. (1988). *The new public health.* Maidenhead, UK: Open University Press.

Berkeley, D., & Springett, J. (2006a). From rhetoric to reality: Barriers faced by Health for All initiatives. *Social Science & Medicine, 63*(1), 179–88. http://dx.doi.org/10.1016/j.socscimed.2005.11.057 Medline:16466835

Berkeley, D., & Springett, J. (2006b). From rhetoric to reality: A systemic approach to understanding the constraints faced by Health For All initiatives in England. *Social Science & Medicine, 63*(11), 2877–89. http://dx.doi.org/10.1016/j.socscimed.2006.07.023 Medline:16962694

Bernier, J., Rock, M., Roy, M., Bujold, R., & Potvin, L. (2006). Structuring an inter-sector research partnership: A negotiated zone. *Sozial- und Präventivmedizin, 51*(6), 335–44. http://dx.doi.org/10.1007/s00038-006-5071-0 Medline:17658136

Bilodeau, A. (2005). Conditions required for successful inter-sectoral collaboration at the local and regional levels. *Promotion & Education, 12* (Suppl 3), 21–2. Medline:16161844

Boutiller, M., Cleverly, S., & Labonte, R. (2000). Community as a setting for health promotion. In B. Poland, L.W. Green, & I. Rootman (Eds.), *Settings for health promotion. Linking theory and practice* (pp. 250–79). Thousand Oaks, CA: Sage.

Borvil, D.A., & Kishchuk, N. (2007). *Démarche-Action Montreal-Nord. Evaluation participative. Rapport final.* Retrieved February 2009 from http://publications.santemontreal.qc.ca/uploads/tx_asssmpublications/978-2-89494-583-4.pdf

Breslow, L. (1999). From disease prevention to health promotion. *JAMA, 281*(11), 1030–3. http://dx.doi.org/10.1001/jama.281.11.1030 Medline: 10086439

Bujold, R. (2001). *Portraits des tables de concertation de quartier à Montréal. Portrait synthèse.* Montreal: Régie régionale de la santé et des services sociaux de Montréal-Centre.

Butler-Jones, D. (2009). Public health science and practice: From fragmentation to alignment. *Canadian Journal of Public Health, 100,* I-1–I-2.

CACIS. (2002). *Partnership framework.* Retrieved February 2009 from http://www.cacis.umontreal.ca/pdf/Partnership.pdf

Callon, M. (1986). Some elements of a sociology of translation: Domestication of scallops and the fishermen of St-Brieux Bay. In J. Law (Ed.), *Power, action and belief: A new sociology of knowledge* (pp. 196–229). London: Routledge.

Callon, M., Lascoume, P., & Barthe, Y. (2001). *Agir dans un monde incertain. Essai sur la démocratie technique.* Paris: Seuil.

Chief Public Health Officer. (2008). *Report on the state of public health in Canada, 2008. Addressing health inequalities.* Ottawa, Ministry of Health.

Direction de la santé publique de Montréal. (1998). *1998 annual report on the health of the population. Social inequalities in health.* Montreal: Régie régionale de la santé et des services sociaux de Montréal-centre. Retrieved February 2009 from http://publications.santemontreal.qc.ca/uploads/tx_asssmpublications/2-89494-122-6.pdf

Direction de la santé publique de Montréal. (2001). Pour une participation effective à l'amélioration de la santé de la population II. Planification stratégique 2001–2004 de la direction de la santé publique de Montréal-Centre: Bilan et perspective. Montreal: Régie régionale de la santé et des services sociaux de Montréal-Centre.

Fassin, D. (1998). Politiques des corps et gouvernement des villes. La production locale de la santé publique. In D. Fassin (Ed.), *Les figures urbaines de la santé publique. Enquêtes sur des expériences locales* (pp. 7–46). Paris: La découverte.

Frohlich, K.L., & Potvin, L. (2008). Transcending the known in public health practice: The inequality paradox. *American Journal of Public Health, 98*(2), 216–21. http://dx.doi.org/10.2105/AJPH.2007.114777 Medline: 18172133

Godbout, J.T. (2000). *Le don, la dette et l'identité: Homo donator versus homo economicus.* Paris: Éditions La Découverte.

Godbout, J.T. (2005). Le marché et le don: Vers une typologie dynamique des liens sociaux. In F. Saillant & E. Gagnon (Eds.), *Communautés et socialités. Formes et force du lien social dans la modernité tardive* (pp. 131–45). Montreal: Liber.

Gouvernement du Québec. (2009). *Mandat: Conférence administrative régionale.* Retrieved February 2009 from http://www.formulaire.gouv.qc.ca/cgi/affiche_doc.cgi?dossier=257&table=0

Hordijk, M., & Baud, I. (2006). The role of research and knowledge generation in collective action and urban governance: How can researchers act as catalysts? *Habitat International, 30*(3), 668–89. http://dx.doi.org/10.1016/j.habitatint.2005.04.002

Kickbusch, I. (2002). Global health governance: Some theoretical considerations on the new political space. In K. Lee (Ed.), *Health impacts of globalization: Towards global governance* (pp. 192–203). London: Palgrave.

Kickbusch, I. (Ed.). (2009). *Policy innovation for health.* New York: Springer. http://dx.doi.org/10.1007/978-0-387-79876-9

Laforest, R., & Phillips, S. (2001). Repenser les relations entre gouvernement et secteur bénévole. *Politique et Sociétés, 20*(2–3), 37–69. http://dx.doi.org/10.7202/040274ar

Laperrière, H., & Zúñiga, R. (2006). Sociopolitical determinants of an AIDS prevention program: Multiple actors and vertical relationships of control and influence. *Policy, Politics & Nursing Practice, 7*(2), 125–35. http://dx.doi.org/10.1177/1527154406289638 Medline:16864636

Latour, B. (2005). *Re-assembling the social. An introduction to Actor-Network Theory.* US: Oxford University Press.

MacKian, S., Elliott, H., Busby, H., & Popay, J. (2003). "Everywhere and nowhere": Locating and understanding the "new" public health. *Health & Place, 9*(3), 219–29. http://dx.doi.org/10.1016/S1353-8292(02)00054-0 Medline:12810329

Mantoura, P., Gendron, S., & Potvin, L. (2007). Participatory research in public health: Creating innovative alliances for health. *Health & Place, 13*(2), 440–51. http://dx.doi.org/10.1016/j.healthplace.2006.05.002 Medline: 16797216

Nelisse, C. (1994). La croisée du formel et de l'informel: Entre l'état et les partenariats. *Lien Social et Politiques—RIAC,* (32): 179–88.

Potvin, L. (2007). Managing uncertainty through participation. In D.M. McQueen, I. Kickbusch, L. Potvin, J. Peilikan, L. Balbo, & T. Abel (Eds.). *Health and modernity. The role of theory in health promotion* (pp. 103–28). New York: Springer.

Potvin, L., Gendron, S., Bilodeau, A., & Chabot, P. (2005). Integrating social theory into public health practice. *American Journal of Public Health, 95*(4), 591–5. http://dx.doi.org/10.2105/AJPH.2004.048017 Medline:15798114

Potvin, L., Hawe, P., & Di Ruggiero, E. (2009). The population health intervention research for Canada. *Canadian Journal of Public Health, 100,* Insert 1.

Potvin, L., Lessard, R., & Fournier, P. (2002). Inégalités sociales de santé. Un partenariat de recherche et de formation. *Canadian Journal of Public Health, 93*(2), 134–7. Medline:11963518

Potvin, L., & McQueen, D.M. (2007). Modernity, public health and health promotion: A reflexive discourse. In D.M. McQueen, I. Kickbusch, L. Potvin, J. Peilikan, L. Balbo, & T. Abel (Eds.), *Health & modernity. The role of theory in health promotion* (pp. 12–20). New York: Springer.

Potvin, L., McQueen, D.V., & Hall, M. (2008). Introduction. Aligning evaluation research and health promotion values: Practices from the Americas. In L. Potvin & D.V. McQueen (Eds.), *Health promotion evaluation practices in the Americas: Values and research* (pp. 1–9). New York: Springer. http://dx.doi.org/10.1007/978-0-387-79733-5_1

Sénécal, G., Herjean, P., Cloutier, G. (2006). *Le quartier comme espace transactionnel.* Montreal: Institut national de recherche scientifique. Retrieved February 2009 from http://www.cacis.umontreal.ca/pdf/rapport-tables.pdf

WHO. (1986). *The Ottawa charter for health promotion.* Retrieved February 2009 from http://www.who.int/healthpromotion/conferences/previous/ottawa/en/print.html

WHO. (2005). *The Bangkok charter for health promotion in a globalised world.* Retrieved February 2009 from http://www.who.int/healthpromotion/conferences/6gchp/bangkok_charter/en/

WHO Commission on Social Determinants of Health. (2008). *Closing the gap in one generation. Health equity through action on the social determinants of health.* Retrieved February 2009 from http://whqlibdoc.who.int/publications/2008/9789241563703_eng.pdf

6 The Back Road from Framework to Policy

LINDA O'BRIEN-PALLAS IN COLLABORATION WITH LAUREEN HAYES

Planning for the efficient and effective delivery of healthcare services to meet the health needs of the populations is a significant challenge. Globally, policy-makers, educators, health service researchers, leaders of unions and professional associations, and other key stakeholders struggle with the best way to build a workforce to fulfil the health needs of populations. To meet this challenge, achieving the appropriate balance between human and non-human resources is important and requires continuous monitoring, careful attention to the country-specific context in which policy decisions are made, and evidence-based decision-making (O'Brien-Pallas, 2002; O'Brien-Pallas, Duffield, Tomblin Murphy, Birch, & Meyer, 2005; O'Brien-Pallas, Tomblin Murphy, Baumann, & Birch, 2001). Many past health human resources (HHR) planning attempts were atheoretical and lacked common databases on which to analyse multiple hypotheses to build the science.

Human resource planning must fall within the broader system in which healthcare services are provided. The effect of social, political, geographical, technological, and economic factors on the efficient and effective mix of human and non-human resources must be considered in planning for, and managing, the healthcare workforce. The issue of political will is also important. Today's human resource challenges have evolved slowly over the past fifty years. Past mistakes cannot be overcome within the time frame of one or even two political mandates. Although critical, it is difficult for policy-makers and key stakeholders to sustain HHR planning efforts, given changing governments and political agendas. Policy-makers and researchers must work in concert to keep health policy issues relevant, easily understood, and practical (O'Brien-Pallas et al., 2005).

The CHSRF/CIHR Chair in Health Human Resources, having received stable funding, can report on measurable outcomes at the end of ten years. Recognition of the need for increased research capacity in nursing management, and for more effective application of new evidence in policy decisions, influenced my chair application. This chair aimed to advance knowledge of HHR science, build research capacity, and work with government and administrative stakeholders in policy development and planning. In this chapter, I describe the development of two models for HHR; one views HHR as a guiding framework at the macro/population level (from our earlier research), and the other, the Patient Care Systems Model, provides theoretical direction at the micro level (O'Brien-Pallas et al., 2003c). I also reflect on the nature of our work with decision-makers in research, knowledge translation, and use of findings, and on my mentorship of students as they began their journeys to becoming independent researchers. Our work and research resulted in information that guided policy decisions. To set the context, I describe the HHR concerns in nursing before my chair, and the Nursing Research Unit's ongoing work to address these concerns.

Open system thinking has driven all of my work. As a high school student I played in my school orchestra. It was there that I first realized the first principle of open system theory – the whole is greater than the sum of its parts. That is, an excellent performance, unless a solo is indicated, requires not one instrument working alone but a group of instruments working together under the direction of an excellent conductor. As I matured as a scientist I was greatly influenced by the work of Bertalanffy (1950; 1967), Jelinek (1967), and Leatt (Leatt et al., 1996; Leatt & Schneck, 1982). Over the years, open systems theory gave me the foundation to examine the interplay between organizational characteristics and system outcomes as it relates to nursing and health services.

Background Context

Nursing Human Resources in the 1990s

In the mid-1990s it seemed as though no one except the nursing community was concerned about the future health and well-being of the nursing workforce and the healthcare needs of the population. As financial pressures grew, there was a trend towards casual labour, deskilling, and just-in-time staffing replacement. Media actively reported layoffs and "casualization" of the nursing workforce in response to downsizing in all health sectors (O'Brien-Pallas & Baumann, 2000). There were growing fears about nurses' health, the outcomes of nurse layoffs, and healthcare system restructuring, as well as the realization that aging baby boomers would constitute a looming resource shortage (O'Brien-Pallas, Alksnis, & Wang, 2003a). The 1990s also saw declining enrolments in nursing schools and fewer new nursing graduates. Nurses who were under thirty years old were increasingly employed in part-time and casual positions, and lacked opportunities to be socialized into the profession and gain the experience they needed to refine their skills.

In teaching hospitals, the number of nursing paid hours per patient day increased, influenced by medical acuity and nursing complexity of patients, compression of patient interventions into a shorter time frame, and the complexity resulting from repeated structural changes in the work environment (O'Brien-Pallas & Baumann, 2000). At that time, researchers were beginning to understand relationships between complex variables and nursing work, but had not developed measurement systems to track the influence on nursing resource use and patient outcomes.

In Canada, it became apparent that unless serious workplace issues were addressed, the physiological and psychological stress in nurses' work environments would accelerate. Older nurses would continue to seek early retirement, mid-career nurses would leave nursing or take part-time hours to have control over the demands of work, and potential nursing applicants would chose alternate careers with more enticing conditions and competitive reimbursement packages. Confounding the situation was the fact that the few individuals who were conducting HHR research would be retiring. Approaches to estimating human resource requirements for nursing were few and plagued with methodological and conceptual limitations. A big challenge was the lack of assessable clinical, administrative, and provider databases that could be linked to conduct complex modelling activities.

The Nursing Research Unit

Within the Nursing Research Unit (NRU), the work being done for the Ontario Ministry of Health and Long-Term Care (MOHLTC) was congruent with the chair's objectives. Since 1991, Dr Andrea Baumann and I co-directed the NRU, which has two sites – one at the University of Toronto under my direction, and one at McMaster University under Baumann's. At its inception, the unit's mandate was to conduct research to expand the understanding of factors that influence the quality of work life for nurses. At the time the HHR chair was awarded, the unit focused on human resource issues in order to investigate restructuring and its impact on the nursing workforce, workforce planning and projection, the nursing shortage, recruitment, retention, and effective use of nurses. In 2004, the unit's revised mandate (under the new name of Nursing Health Services Research Unit) has reflected a broadened scope of research ranging from the new graduate to the late career nurse, and covering community, hospital, and long-term care settings.

Prior to the beginning of my chair, the NRU had been instrumental to the work of the Nursing Task Force in Ontario (Nursing Task Force, 1999). In September 1998, Minister of Health Elizabeth Witmer established a task force to examine nursing services in Ontario, to identify how changes in the profession affected the delivery of healthcare services, and to recommend how the province's health system could be improved through nursing services. The Nursing Task Force recommended that the Joint Provincial Nursing Committee (JPNC) monitor the implementation of the recommendations and evaluate their effectiveness. The JPNC is a joint committee of key nursing stakeholder organizations and the MOHLTC that provides advice on health reform from a nursing perspective and supports communication between nursing groups and the government. The JPNC and its working groups receive administrative and policy support from the Nursing Secretariat, a division of the MOHLTC created in 1999 to provide advice on healthcare and public policy from a nursing perspective (Joint Provincial Nursing Committee, 2001).

Beginning the Chair Journey

An *Environmental Scan on Health Services Research Priorities* (Canadian Policy Research Networks, 2001) identified HHR as a key priority for health services research, with a focus on recruitment, retention, quality of the workplace, and planning models. The CHSRF/CIHR Chair in Nursing Health Human Resources was created to positively impact the HHR situation by developing an applied research capacity and improving the linkages and exchanges within the health system. A ten-year horizon was seen as sufficient to build applied research capacity towards resolving the methodological challenges of determining how many nurses (and allied health personnel) are required to meet current and future client, nursing, and health system needs.

The chair would address the challenges of bringing together the participation of many actors in the health system, aiming to improve the availability and reliability of research findings and ensure policy-makers can understand and use them. The goal was to develop a critical mass of practitioners in policy and administrative settings to foster communication among policy-makers, administrative partners, and academics conducting HHR research. The HHR framework would be applied to advance HHR science and guide planning and policy, bringing evidence to the decision-making process. As it was, there was too little policy on the development and effective management of nursing resources. Building on the work already underway with the Nursing Task Force in Ontario, I believed the chair would make my contribution more effective at both the provincial and national levels. In the absence of the chair award, I still planned to research HHR in nursing, but a heavier teaching load and fewer resources would have limited my influence over policy and planning.

In essence, the chair would provide a vehicle to begin to avert the nursing crisis and its impact on the health system. The HHR chair's program objectives were as follows: (1) further develop and validate a model to estimate future nurse resource requirements and examine the impact of HHR decisions on population, provider, and system outcomes; (2) identify management strategies that can be used to reduce nurses' physical and psychological strain and improve health outcomes of nurses; (3) provide education and mentorship opportunities for multidisciplinary health system researchers and stakeholders; (4) liaise with provincial, national, and international policy- and decision-makers and with the JPNC; and (5) develop a communication and knowledge transfer strategy at the local, national, and international level. While these goals were ambitious, I saw the required activities as interconnected. For example, studies being conducted within the chair's program would act as a tool to build capacity in students through developing research expertise and laying the foundation for new relationships between researchers and policy-makers.

Ongoing affiliation with the MOHLTC, the decision-making partner for the HHR chair, was already established in the research processes under the NRU. The NRU conducted research to inform evidence-based policy and management decisions related to health and nursing services and to develop a joint mechanism for knowledge transfer. These aims matched the chair's objectives closely and would help me answer required research questions and build capacity for the future. The chair would continue to lead multidisciplinary teams to help solve the complex HHR issues and guide and mentor doctoral and postdoctoral students to sustain applied research capacity in the future. At the time, each of my doctoral, postdoctoral, and other students was actively engaged in the NRU. The chair would also sit on MOHLTC multidisciplinary committees associated with HHR to provide a mechanism for research transfer and use in developing nursing and allied health HHR policy.

The Development of Models for HHR

The HHR Conceptual Framework

A major focus of the chair was to advance the underdeveloped science of HHR planning. Two of my colleagues were particularly instrumental in the development of an HHR conceptual framework: Stephen Birch, a professor from the Department of Clinical Epidemiology and Biostatistics at McMaster University; and Gail Tomblin Murphy, a professor of nursing at Dalhousie University. HHR planning has traditionally been supply driven, based on the assumptions that structure alone determines the service needs of the population. The main limitation of this approach is its failure to reflect the complex nature of the processes underlying the needs for services (population health) and the delivery of services (healthcare provision), as well as the effects of HHR planning on population, provider, and system outcomes (Birch, O'Brien-Pallas, Alksnis, Tomblin Murphy, & Thomson, 2003).

We emphasized that HHR requirements should be considered along with the levels and mix of resources used to produce healthcare services. Resource requirements are impacted by demand factors including population demographics, innovations and technology, availability of treatment options, access to services, service use, and incidence of disease (Birch et al., 2003). However, one of the key challenges to estimating human resource requirements for nursing has been the lack of accessible clinical, administrative, and provider databases for complex modelling activities. The conceptual inadequacy of the models and the use of simple supply models have contributed to numerous swings between shortages and surpluses of nurses noted internationally, even

Figure 6.1 Health System and Human Resources Planning Conceptual Framework

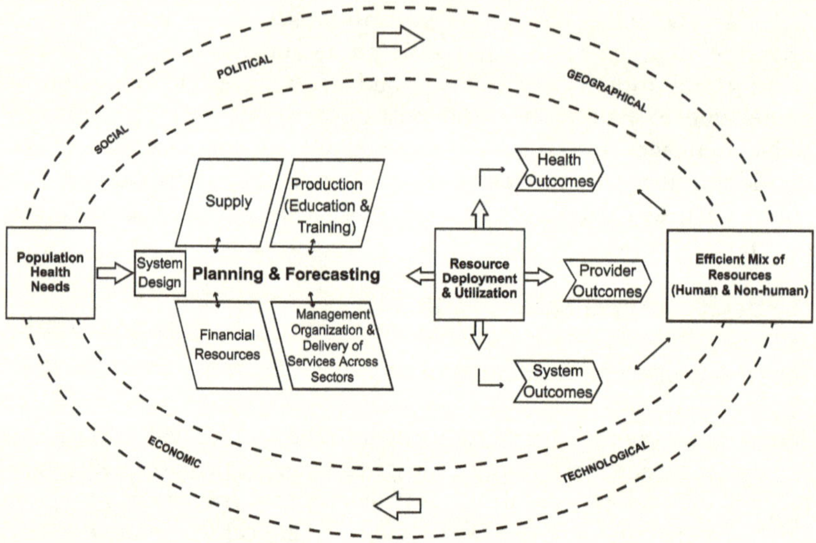

Source: O'Brien-Pallas, Tomblin Murphy, Baumann, & Birch, 2001 (adapted from O'Brien-Pallas & Baumann, 1997).

though policy-makers identified HHR as a major priority for health services research.

The health system and human resources planning conceptual framework (Figure 6.1), developed by O'Brien-Pallas, Tomblin Murphy, Baumann, and Birch (2001), is an adaptation of earlier work (O'Brien-Pallas & Baumann, 1997). At the core of the framework is the recognition that health human resources must match the health needs of the population as closely as possible. The elements of the framework that highlight the complexity and dynamic nature of HHR planning include: population health needs; supply of providers; production (education and training); financial resources; management, organization, and delivery of health services; resource deployment and use; population health outcomes; system outcomes; and efficient and effective mix of human resources (O'Brien-Pallas, 2002).

Developing and validating a conceptual framework for HHR planning was a founding goal of the chair program and a key deliverable, having been applied in the work of national and international organizations such as the Canadian Institute of Health Information (CIHI) and the World Health Organization (WHO). The CIHI report *Guidance Document for the Development of Data Sets to Support Health Human Resources Management in Canada* (Tomblin Murphy & O'Brien-Pallas, 2005) consisted of a consultation process to identify and validate HHR priority information needs and indicators, as well as to identify standard data elements to collect across Canada. My work with the WHO Global Alliance for Nursing and Midwifery involved monitoring progress within WHO member states in relation to five key areas (human resources planning, management, education, practice, and leadership) based on standardized indicators.

The Patient Care Systems Model

While the HHR framework applies at the population/macro level, the patient care delivery model (PCDM) was used in our research to identify strategies to improve outcomes of nurses, patients, and the care delivery system. Providing theoretical direction at the micro level, the patient care delivery model (Figure 6.2) builds on previous work by Jelinek (1967) who discusses a patient care system as composed of input (i.e., resources) and output factors. He describes a transformation of inputs into outputs that was influenced by workload, organizational, and environmental factors. The PCDM expands Jelinek's model and exemplifies the application of Bertalanffy's (1950) general systems theory (GST) to a healthcare organization. The PCDM conceptualizes the delivery of nursing services on patient care units, which are production subsystems within the larger hospital system.

Input factors comprise characteristics of patients, nurses, and the system, as well as system unit behaviours. Such behaviours include organizational practices related to nurse staffing assignments, continuity of care, and the division of work. The PCDM highlights the interdependence and interaction between patient, nurse, work environment, and system factors, which in turn influence outcomes. Outputs include changes in patient health status; nurse employment outcomes; and system efficiency, quality, and staffing stability. These outputs provide feedback to the system itself because positive outcomes ensure that members of the community continue to use the organization's services, staff are retained to provide the services, and the organization's accreditation and funding are sustained.

Figure 6.2 Patient Care Delivery Model

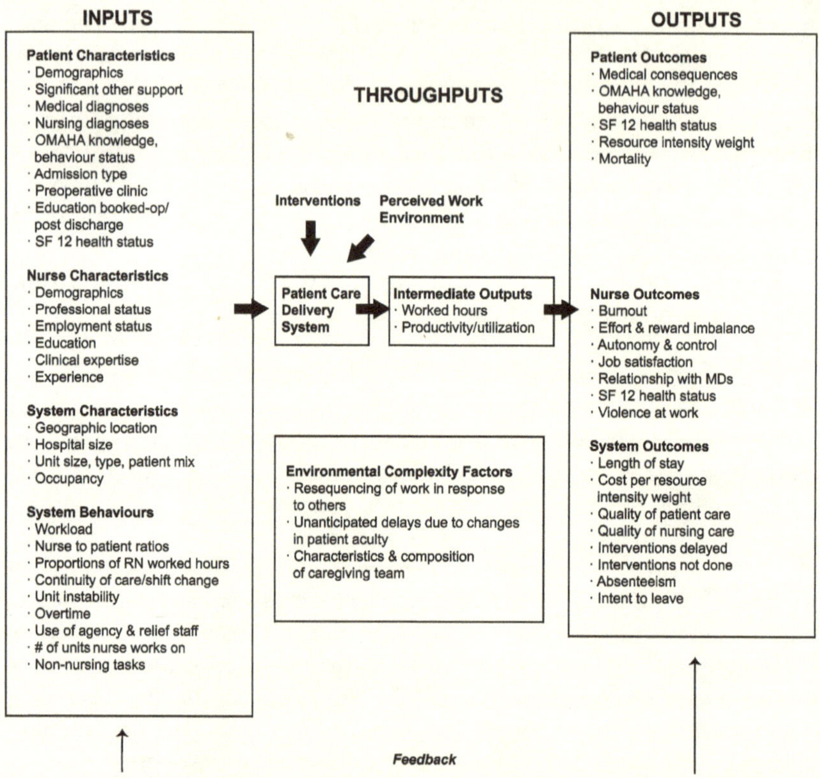

Source: O'Brien-Pallas et al., 2003c.

Research Findings and Key Messages

Advancing HHR science has been achieved through several research grants to advance the understanding of key elements within the HHR framework. At the macro level, HHR simulation helps determine the number and types of personnel, and the types of educational programs, required to meet future needs. The micro level involves estimating the number and type of nursing personnel required on a daily basis to achieve client, provider, and systems outcomes. Decision-makers and nursing administrators often rely on simple supply and demand approaches for macro level estimates, and on counting nursing tasks to determine the number of nurses needed during the next shift for micro level estimates. I will now highlight some research findings and key messages resulting from the research that contribute to a better insight of the HHR issues that policy-makers face and the implications decision-makers must consider.

HHR Planning

Validation of the HHR framework as a research outcome was an important part of the chair's research platform. As her dissertation study, one of my former doctoral students developed and tested a way to establish, monitor, and predict needs for nursing services by using the health needs of the population (Tomblin Murphy, 2005). Her findings demonstrated that it is possible to model needs for nursing HHR based on the health needs of the population and apply the modelling to nursing services policies and planning at the population level.

Our research study, *Health Human Resource Modelling: Challenging the Past, Creating the Future* (O'Brien-Pallas et al., 2007), further validated the HHR conceptual framework and addressed the dynamic nature of the needs for, and provision and management of, nursing human resources. Our findings emphasized that HHR planning should not assume that healthcare needs in the population remain constant; changes in population health needs over time are complex and vary depending on the indicator used. To model such changes requires consistently measured indicators collected through periodic population health surveys. In terms of needed nursing services, the required number of nurses to deliver a planned level of service (or manage a particular patient mix) depends on the configuration of hospital inputs that are context-specific and on the methods of production. Plans to change other inputs (e.g., number of beds) must consider implications for nurse human resource requirements to achieve desired levels of services.

At the macro level, HHR simulations help determine the number and types of personnel, and the types of educational programs, required to meet future needs. The HHR framework has been used in planning exercises undertaken for Atlantic Canada, in which researchers consolidated available data and developed a scenario-based HHR simulation model (Birch et al., 2005). Such simulations provide information about the impact of different policies, creating the opportunity for a policy portfolio that aims to match policies with the nature of the underlying problems and avoid time lags in responsiveness to current problems (see Birch et al., 2007). We hope to see more use of HHR simulations to better apply theoretical principles to HHR policy development.

Staffing Stability

HHR planning within organizations requires daily estimates of the number and type of nursing personnel needed to achieve client, provider, and systems outcomes. Ensuring the staffing can meet workload demands can enhance quality of care. One of the most important policy issues relates to nursing turnover. Our research, *Understanding the Costs and Outcomes of Nurses' Turnover in Canadian Hospitals,* shows that turnover of nurses is a major problem and is accompanied by temporary replacement costs and initial lower productivity of new hires (O'Brien-Pallas et al., 2008). Therefore, nurse turnover should be monitored in all types of delivery systems and the variables contributing to turnover should be clearly defined and measured across sectors.

Our research indicates that retention strategies should address the physical and mental health of nurses, the balance of efforts and rewards associated with work, nurse autonomy, the full scope of practice, managerial relationships, innovative work schedules, more full-time permanent positions, and reasonable nurse-patient ratios based on targeted productivity standards. Attention to these areas will minimize the effect of persistently high job demands and reduce absenteeism and overtime. Our findings suggest that retention is more likely when nurses have job security, the ability to work to their full scope of practice, and an appropriate workload. The probability of medical error is also reduced when turnover is controlled.

Appropriate Workload

Our research underscores the need to implement effective and efficient mechanisms to address workload issues. The evidenced-based staffing study (O'Brien-Pallas et al., 2003c) tested the patient care delivery model and provided new empirical evidence of the link between nurse staffing (i.e., use) levels, patient and provider outcomes, and system effectiveness. Maximum productivity is 93 per cent, as 7 per cent of the shift is made up of mandatory paid breaks. However, we recommended that nursing unit productivity target 85 per cent, plus or minus 5 per cent, as levels higher than this lead to higher costs, poorer patient care, and poorer nurse outcomes. Above a particular threshold of nursing unit use (i.e., the proportion of nurse hours worked relative to patient workload), we observed lower levels of patient outcomes (e.g., declines in patient health status and behaviours) and system outcomes (e.g., longer than expected length of stay). Therefore, we suggest challenging decision-makers to maximize productivity and minimize staffing costs, while ensuring the quality of care.

Competent and Knowledgeable Nurses

Ensuring that nurses have the required knowledge and skills is critical to quality work environments and positive outcomes. Our research, "Evaluation of a client care delivery model: Variability in client outcomes in community home nursing" (O'Brien-Pallas et al., 2002) provided supporting evidence in Ontario's move towards the baccalaureate entry to practice in nursing. The findings revealed: "For every unit increase in assignment of baccalaureate-prepared nurses, clients will on average demonstrate an 80 per cent greater likelihood of improvement in knowledge scores and a 120 per cent greater likelihood of improvement in behaviour scores in relation to their health condition at discharge" (O'Brien-Pallas et al., 2002). A few years later, we again demonstrated a relationship between baccalaureate nursing education and improved patient outcomes, this time in the hospital setting (O'Brien-Pallas et al., 2003c).

Healthy and Professional Work Environment

Our research consistently shows that work environments should promote nurse health and support professional development. Enhancing nurse autonomy, reducing emotional exhaustion, and having enough staff to cope with rapidly changing patient conditions can help meet productivity targets. Resources should be in place and tools available to optimize nurses' competencies and allow them to work to their full scope of practice and provide effective care. Good quality care comes from considering patient safety, training health professionals to match patient acuity, and knowing about each other's responsibilities to promote collegial working relationships. An appropriate skill mix, clear roles for team members, and effective communication across caregiver groups are important, as they reduce role ambiguity and conflict. Our research also highlights the importance of effective leadership at all levels of healthcare organizations in providing supportive practice settings. Leadership is pivotal to reducing nurse turnover as it helps address its underlying factors.

Improved Databases

To ensure appropriate allocation of nursing resources and advancement of HHR planning beyond simple supply and demand forecasting, investment is needed to create and maintain readily accessible databases that allow comparison between and among jurisdictions. Policy options must be informed by good quality, comparable, and readily accessible evidence. Linking data from a broad range of areas in organizations requires a sustainable investment in data and capacity building. Investment is also needed for infrastructure, so that researchers may collect data that enhance monitoring and improve care delivery and measurement of performance outcomes. Data that should be routinely captured include valid workload measurement; environmental complexity; patient nursing diagnoses and ratings of knowledge, behaviour, and status; nurse and patient health status; nurse-to-patient ratios; and productivity. More consistent and standardized reporting of information that relates to the model elements is needed at both macro and micro levels. More available administrative databases would facilitate better research with improved data collection and analysis of relationships between the input factors and outcomes, such as how nurse staffing decisions influence outcomes.

Education and Mentorship

The chair award made it possible for me to supervise more students and provide greater latitude with regard to funding support for those students than I would have been able to otherwise. Doctoral fellowships allowed students to focus on their doctoral coursework and theses. Postdoctoral fellowships exposed students to research studies already in progress as well as time and tutoring in submitting new grant applications. We also implemented the six-month Chair Research Apprenticeship offered to health service administrators, policy-makers, planners, and nurses who wished to develop expertise in HHR research. The apprentices developed learning objectives in combination with their employers with the aim to help enhance research capacity in their home organizations after completing the apprenticeship.

Field placements at the NRU facilitated the study goals of the chair participants. This setting enabled participants to actively participate in actual research projects, to network with researchers nationally and internationally, and to access in-house statisticians and infrastructure support such as reserved desk space and computers. My connections with government leaders and policy-makers allowed trainees to link with relevant experts and opportunities.

I strive to apply leadership principles advocated by Kouzes and Posner (1997) in my day-to-day mentorship. "Modelling the way" involves working alongside a team, particularly when the going gets rough. Very early on, I understood that I could not ask a team member or a student to do something I was not prepared to do myself. Involving young scientists in discussions with decision-makers, especially when decision-makers are not keen to hear the research findings is another important modelling behaviour. In doing this, young scientists can observe the need for diplomacy coupled with dead honesty in conveying a research message. They can also critique the process and identify strategies for improving communication in future situations. Modelling helps new researchers learn from a mentor's experiences and visualize themselves in similar situations as they mentally practice for future opportunities. "Enabling others," another strategy Kouzes and Posner discuss, involves mentoring with a special focus on helping an individual feel they can achieve what seems impossible. Every doctoral student recalls the time when completing their thesis requirements seemed just out of reach. As chair, I have learned that enabling others also requires exposing and linking young scientists to opportunities where their talent and expertise can be recognized, and letting go of the spotlight so that others can flourish.

Along with the annual reporting requirements for the chair, I regularly include testimonial letters that express students' views of their relevant learning. Some of their statements relate to specific learning, such as improving statistical skills by running and interpreting statistical analyses with the assistance of the senior research associate using SPSS software. Others make general reference developing research skills and gaining practical experience with research projects. The following are some of my students' statements:

- I have not only gained confidence in the management of research projects but have also gained research experience, which enhances the potential for my involvement in other research.

- [This program] has also promoted my learning and development in the field of research by involving me in the preparation and submission of research grant proposals.
- Opportunities have been very helpful in enabling me to interact with key nursing and policy leaders and to discuss and debate current issues and trends.
- Research such as the Evidence Based Staffing Study, the Nursing Sector Study, and the soon-to-be released Turnover Study provide me with key facts and evidence that I am able to use in my health authority to influence decision-making.
- [This program] has provided opportunities for me to learn about how research is conducted and how to collaborate with stakeholders before, during, and after research projects.
- I have valued the opportunities to be involved with the research projects at the Nursing Health Services Research Unit and know that I have grown personally and professionally because of these opportunities.
- This apprenticeship was a unique opportunity to learn the research process from a very practical perspective and then to be able to transfer the knowledge and skill back into the practice setting.

In addition, two of my doctoral students used or adapted the patient care delivery model in their studies, which included an examination of the work environment and medication errors in paediatric hospitals (Sears, 2009) and leadership practices and outcomes in adult hospitals in Saskatchewan (Eisler, 2009). Such testimonies demonstrate the value of research activities as a platform to link and mentor decision-makers and researchers, thereby contributing to capacity building for future generations.

Planning and arranging positive learning opportunities is a challenging task. An obstacle we encountered was the difficulty in attracting and supporting participants from outside Toronto. An actual presence in the NRU enriched the learning experiences, and so it was important to accommodate on-site time for chair participants. To overcome the challenge of geography, we adapted residency periods and added a distance option facilitated by email and teleconferences. On-site residencies were possible with employers' support, as salary replacement funding covered travel and accommodation costs. Also, the number of placements the chair could support was limited; therefore, we formed a partnership with the University of Toronto's Health Network, which provided annual funding support for the research apprenticeship positions.

Linkage and Exchange

Linkage and exchange is both a philosophy and a set of activities and is a central thread in the chair's research, teaching, and knowledge dissemination. The chair's activities involving mentorship are integrated with linkage and exchange, as I include my graduate students in the collaboration with our decision-maker partners. Although one of the chair's objectives is to promote greater use of research findings, policy-makers are required to weigh research-based facts along with several other factors to determine action. Policy-makers have struggled with how to use evidence to guide decisions when evidence is sparse and the political fallout from one course of action over another is significant (O'Brien-Pallas, 2003). Even with compelling research findings, the chair's government stakeholders still considered the values of society, competing priorities, and pressure from the public, media, and other interest groups in their decision-making processes (O'Brien-Pallas & Baumann, 2000).

To keep our research in the forefront, I have tried to ensure that important findings relating to nursing health human resources are shared in a timely manner with key groups and individuals, both within the MOHLTC and abroad. Several times each year, I participate in conferences and consultations nationally and internationally. My work with the WHO has required frequent trips to Geneva. Most years I have travelled with colleagues to the International Conference of Nurses and Sigma Theta Tau International.

Since the beginning of my chair, I have sought out other decision-making partners. One of these is the chair of my advisory committee, Tom Closson, who was CEO and president of the University of Toronto's Health Network at the time. The chair's advisory committee is multidisciplinary and composed of experts and stakeholders who meet with me twice a year and provide guidance and expertise. The chair's advisory members have facilitated the implementation of the chair's program in various ways, including providing communication expertise and offering input into overall strategic planning. For example, the advisory committee was very helpful in providing direction for media appearances (television and radio), profiling the chair at meetings of the Canadian Association of Schools of Nursing and the Council of Ontario Universities, and facilitating development of the chair website.

While linkage and exchange activities are vital to my research program, they involve some ongoing challenges. Jonathan Lomas (2000, p. 239) highlighted some issues in linkage and exchange in research environments and decision-making organizations:

- Time: not enough, given workloads; finding commonly available time to meet;
- Timelines: not enough lead time from funding agency for development of linkage; decision-makers often need results faster than the research process can produce them;
- Multiple decision-maker partners: resource-intensive to tailor a project to the (sometimes competing) needs and agendas of multiple decision-maker partners;
- Finding decision-makers: no obvious or single point of entry into decision-maker organizations; broad array of potential partners with no way of knowing which ones are influential;
- Moving targets: frequent personnel changes, which discourage investment of time to establish linkage; frequent restructuring which makes it difficult to find stable areas for evaluation.

These challenges match what we, the chair's collaborators and I, have experienced over the years. As most of the day-to-day work within the research unit was under my direction, I can attest to the challenges relating to lack of time. Often the onus is on research staff to arrange team meetings – not an easy task given the full schedules and role overload typical of most investigators. Also, lack of time made it difficult for us to efficiently report our findings in peer-reviewed journals, usually due to ongoing competing demands. However, our publications have been successful, and I began to dedicate more time to them in the later part of my chair.

As researchers, we are acutely aware that decision-making organizations have their own challenges. Having the time to become involved in research is an issue for decision-makers, who do not always understand what is involved in the research process, and do not always have the opportunity to learn. Lomas (2000) refers to the different cultures that surround those who conduct research and those who might be able to use it. Decision-makers might claim that researchers produce irrelevant, poorly communicated products and, in turn, researchers might accuse decision-makers of political expediency that results in irrational outcomes. Thus it is important to bring researchers into the policy-making process to increase consensus and resolve conflict. If decision-makers are to use the research-derived evidence, they need first-hand knowledge of the issues, the research process, and the limitations of HHR research. They also need to be aware of existing research and participate in planning future research (Lomas, 2000).

My work within the chair's program has involved ongoing collaboration with the MOHLTC, which is the primary decision-making partner for the chair. Provincial cabinet shuffles have resulted in changing priorities that the program had to consider in the development of proposals for research funding and building new relationships within the ministry. Maintaining positive collaboration requires clear two-way communication and clear expectations when planning research. There is a process in place for deciding the priority questions to be addressed in the ministry-directed projects.

In the world of research, completing the study is just the first step; making the research come alive and using it to build capacity for future science and scientists, and to tell stories that capture policy-makers' attention and ultimately lead to change, are an ongoing priority (O'Brien-Pallas, 2003, p. 28). In the academic research world, where success is measured by the number of grants won and publications accepted, the broader public good of the research may get lost. Ensuring the adequacy of nursing numbers and creating work environments in which nurses can provide optimal care for patients are the goals that have always guided the chair's research. Our team has used evidence to communicate how excessive workload influences nurses' health, patient outcomes, and healthcare costs. Lavis (2006) states that public policy-making processes are less linear, more unpredictable, and faster-paced than research. Yet substantive policy changes on nursing work are limited and slow to come, even though we have shared evidence. Our team of decision-makers, students, and researchers learned to find excitement in each small step, and this has sustained us for the greater purpose. Celebrating small successes has been the driving force that allowed each of us to recommit to the process of achieving the larger vision.

Added Value of the Chair

I am confident that the chair's support has added value to my professional achievements in many ways. The chair appointment has led to significant recognition of my work and achievements in HHR research, which has brought me credibility and opened the door for membership on high-level committees. Having the opportunity to contribute to the Romanow Commission near the beginning of the chair was exciting, as my role was visible and the commission recognized HHR planning as crucial to the future of Canadian healthcare. In 2002, Gail Tomblin Murphy (one of my doctoral students at the time) and I submitted a discussion paper highlighting the need to redesign work environments for health professionals; increase the use of nurse practitioners in primary healthcare; apply an integrated approach to educational programming for health professionals; invest in creating and maintaining readily accessible databases; and foster solid links between the research and policy communities to move HHR policy-relevant research forward and enhance the use of findings in policy decision-making (Tomblin Murphy & O'Brien-Pallas, 2002). For the commission, I also received an invitation to participate in a panel discussion as part of a series of televised, on-campus policy dialogue sessions to broaden public awareness on key issues in the healthcare system, and to engage national and local experts with a range of perspectives in debate about the potential courses of action. Indeed, I will always remember having a voice in shaping the future of our healthcare system as a high point.

I believe my interactions with the MOHLTC have influenced the use of research results in policy. The chair's involvement with the JPNC ultimately led to a stronger nursing profession, in that nurses have been able to voice areas of concern and facilitate the emergence of some positive trends. With the current shortage of nurses, HHR planning has become an area of interest in Canada, and there have been increased investments made by governments and employers since the early part of this decade. For example, the creation of the nursing strategy resulted in funding allocation to initiatives including late career nurse strategies, new graduate mentorship strategies, clinical simulation equipment for nursing schools, full-time nursing positions, ceiling lifts to improve nurse and patient safety, and nurse practitioner positions. I believe the chair had a positive influence in these changes by contributing to the collective work that underpinned important initiatives.

I believe the chair has contributed towards accomplishments that would have otherwise taken longer. The HHR modelling consultation I provided to the Atlantic Provinces contributed to a multidisciplinary simulation model that tests the effectiveness of policy scenarios before deciding to implement them. Also, I believe my chair facilitated the completion of the national Nursing Sector Study, as it helped me negotiate consensus on recommendations among the many diverse study stakeholders. Completion of the Nursing Sector Study Phase I (Nursing Sector Study Corporation, 2005), in turn, provided the foundation for the development of a pan-Canadian nursing human resource strategy (Phase II) in consultation with government and non-government stakeholders (Nursing Sector Study Corporation, 2006). The Nursing Sector Study provided a better understanding of nursing human resource issues on which to build in our subsequent research.

The chair award has enabled me to participate in national and international events that I otherwise might not have been able to attend. I was invited to a federal health council HHR summit in Toronto, where I spoke to the Members of Parliament about the policy implications of the Nursing Sector Study in Canada. I also attended a high-level international meeting of twenty-three HHR researchers held at the Rockefeller Centre in Bellagio, Italy, which led to a worldwide collective that continues to work on the issue of nurse migration. I have worked with the WHO and the International Council of Nurses as an expert in human resources, and wrote invited papers and sat on working groups and panels. In 2005, I prepared a paper with colleagues on HHR, *Mapping the Policy Trail,* for the International Council of Nurses and participated in a high-level consultation in Geneva with experts from other countries. Linkage and exchange activities have been central to the chair in my efforts to work with decision-makers, make media appearances and presentations, and grow my record of publications.

I believe that my team's research would not have reached such an international scope without the chair support. My involvement with colleagues from other countries has influenced replication of research in their homeland. The Evidence Based Staffing Study was completed in New South Wales, Australia. That team, along with another in New Zealand, replicated the Nursing Turnover Study. Much of my international research has been with the WHO. The chair's team established a global baseline within five key areas (human resources planning, management, education, practice, and leadership) based on standardized indicators, and then monitored changes to this baseline in 2008.

We tracked progress and evaluated the impact of country interventions to improve nursing and midwifery services, considering policy recommendations in *Nursing Midwifery Services: Strategic Directions 2002–2008* and the goals set out in resolutions WHA 54.12 and WHA 59.27 (World Health Organization, 2002). This report assisted WHO and member states to prepare reports for the WHO assembly in 2010.

I believe the chair has added value to education and mentorship that deal with building research capacity. I have been able to expand the number of doctoral and postdoctoral students I supervise, and have offered research opportunities for research associates through the chair funding and support. Research apprentice positions have contributed to better research and evidence-based decision-making in participants' home organizations. Students have also benefited from the regional training centre funding and activities such as the summer institute that my students glowingly described above. The opportunity for these students to be exposed to high-level thinkers and different disciplines involved in the training centres through courses and practicum will enhance their overall learning and build future networks for interdisciplinary research. I have enjoyed assisting the development of the training centres and the annual policy seminars. The chairs' and training centres' regular meetings have provided a way to understand the emerging nature of the CADRE activities. Interacting with the other chairs has been helpful because, while our implementation issues may be different, the sense of belonging and sharing of ideas has benefitted all involved.

The chair has also raised awareness of the need for healthy workplaces for nurses and other healthcare workers through the establishment of the Chair Achievement Award, which recognizes individuals who have used the research evidence and best practices. The chair held symposiums at which researchers and policy-makers shared their HHR knowledge and expertise. Also, I facilitated the creation of the Dorothy M. Wylie Nursing Leadership Institute, a highly specialized and interactive learning experience to mirror the best leadership courses available (Simpson et al., 2002). The chair supported this initiative by allowing (potential) nurse leaders to attend and, for several institutes I held, teaching sessions relating to the nursing work environment. Other senior faculty at the Lawrence S. Bloomberg Faculty of Nursing have now taken up this teaching activity.

In Ontario, the trend of employers laying off and reducing the hours of nurses in attempts to balance their budgets has received media attention. However, significant progress has been made in cultivating the critical mass of practitioners and future researchers who are knowledgeable about nursing HHR issues in the policy and administrative practice settings. We believe that the status of the nursing profession must be taken into account at the highest levels, and the issues nurses face today must be given attention reflected in the government's decisions.

Conclusion

One of the key leverages for chair holders is the opportunity to bring evidence to the decision-making process as we confront and work our way through the potentially alarming shortage of nurses. At the onset of my chair experience, more studies were being conducted to examine the work-life issues facing nursing, but such work was primarily descriptive in nature. While many nurse leaders had attempted to create healthy work environments, inconsistent funding practices made them nearly impossible to sustain. Policy and health planners and nursing administrators relied on simple supply and demand approaches in addressing macro-level HHR estimates, and counting individual tasks to estimate numbers of nurses required for the next shift at the micro level. The chair has supported cutting-edge research to provide estimates of the numbers and types of nursing human resources required to meet predetermined outcomes, develop evidence-based interventions to improve nurses' health and satisfaction, and collaborate with international research projects and exchanges to reduce the worldwide impact of this crisis and learn lessons that can be adapted to the Canadian environment.

The chair has built ongoing linkages and exchanges with its MOHLTC partner to communicate research findings and ensure their application in practice and policy. My close working relations with the senior nursing officials at the national and provincial level, and my membership on the JPNC, allowed me to bring evidence and its interpretation to arenas where policy is developed and recommended to bureaucratic and political officials and to nursing and healthcare organizations. In addition, working closely with nursing unions, professional associations, and influential others has promoted transfer and uptake of research findings and chair activities, and provided real feedback from the field. The combination of these activities has contributed to a critical mass of policy-makers and planners, nurse administrators, and researchers with developed networks to help stabilize the nursing human resource situation and reduce the repetitive cycles of shortage and surpluses of nurses in Canada and worldwide.

In closing, the inaugural CHSRF/CIHR Chair in Nursing Health Human Resources presented two possible scenarios for nursing human resources in 2010. In the first scenario, robot nurses care for patients because there are not enough human nurses to meet the nursing needs of the public, and governments claim they did not know about the severity of the shortage before it became a reality. In the second scenario, the chair has built a strong program to determine the number and type of nurses needed in the new millennium, identified mechanisms to educate them, and researched and disseminated strategies that enabled healthcare employers to create healthy workplaces and excel in recruiting and retaining nurses. I believe the HHR chair contributed to a more robust nursing workforce through ongoing research, which will in turn promote application of HHR planning methods and foster a broad understanding of HHR issues and solutions.

While this chair was seen as a vehicle to help address the nursing crisis in the health system, I believe the work must continue after the chair's funding is terminated, perhaps through another role of similar nature. The success of the HHR chair will ultimately be judged by whether people who need healthcare feel the cold touch of a robotic arm or the caring warmth of a human hand. Use of research findings in HHR policy will result in a more effective healthcare system in the coming years and decades. At the inception of the chair, the Canadian economy was recovering from one recession, and at the end we are in a global recession and face a nursing shortage. The true test of the chair's impact will be the extent to which fiscal decisions are influenced by immediate pressures or by the evidence. Whatever choices are made, this chair and its collaborators have demonstrated the outcomes of such decisions on patients, providers, and the health system.

REFERENCES

Bertalanffy, L. von. (1950). An outline of general system theory. *British Journal for the Philosophy of Science*, *1*(2), 134–65. http://dx.doi.org/10.1093/bjps/I.2.134

Bertalanffy, L. von. (1967). General theory of systems: Application to psychology. *Social Sciences Information. Information Sur les Sciences Sociales*, *6*(6), 125–36. http://dx.doi.org/10.1177/053901846700600610

Birch, S., Kephart, G., O'Brien-Pallas, L., & Tomblin Murphy, G. (2005). *Atlantic Health Human Resources Planning Study*. Submitted to Atlantic Health Human Resources Association. Submitted by Med-Emerg Inc. Executive summary (pp. 1–25). Retrieved on 18 February 2013 from http://www.nlhba.nl.ca/hr/documents/Full%20Report.pdf

Birch, S., Kephart, G., Tomblin Murphy, G., O'Brien-Pallas, L., Alder, R., & MacKenzie, A. (2007). Human resources planning and the production of health: A needs-based analytical framework. *Canadian Public Policy, 33*(s1), 1–16. http://dx.doi.org/10.3138/9R62-Q0V1-L188-1406

Birch, S., O'Brien-Pallas, L., Alksnis, C., Tomblin Murphy, G.T., & Thomson, D. (2003). Beyond demographic change in human resources planning: An extended framework and application to nursing. *Journal of Health Services Research & Policy, 8*(4), 225–9. http://dx.doi.org/10.1258/135581903322403290 Medline:14596757

Canadian Policy Research Networks. (2001). *Environmental scan on health services research priorities*. Retrieved on 18 February 2013 from http://www.cfhi-fcass.ca/Libraries/Listening_for_Direction/LfD_I_environmental_scan_e.sflb.ashx

Eisler, K. (2009). *The leadership practices of nurse managers and the association with nursing staff retention and the promotion of quality care in two Saskatchewan hospitals*. Thesis (PhD), University of Toronto, 2009. Retrieved from http://hdl.handle.net/1807/17459

Jelinek, R.C. (1967). A structural model for the patient care operation. *Health Services Research, 2*(3), 226–42. Medline:6081241

Joint Provincial Nursing Committee. (2001). *Good nursing, good health: A good investment*. Progress Report on the Nursing Task Force Strategy in Ontario. Retrieved on 18 February 2013 from http://www.health.gov.on.ca/en/common/ministry/publications/reports/nurserep01/616209_moh_good_nursing.pdf

Kouzes, J., & Posner, B. (1997). *The leadership challenge: How to keep getting extraordinary things done in organizations*. San Francisco, CA: Jossey-Bass Publishing.

Lavis, J.N. (2006). Research, public policymaking, and knowledge-translation processes: Canadian efforts to build bridges. *The Journal of Continuing Education in the Health Professions, 26*(1), 37–45. http://dx.doi.org/10.1002/chp.49 Medline:16557509

Leatt, P., Pink, G.H., & Naylor, C.D. (1996). Integrated delivery systems: Has their time come in Canada? *Canadian Medical Association Journal, 154*(6), 803–9. Medline:8634958

Leatt, P., & Schneck, R. (1982). Work environments of different types of nursing subunits. *Journal of Advanced Nursing*, *7*(6), 581–94. http://dx.doi.org/10.1111/j.1365-2648.1982.tb00279.x Medline:6924944

Lomas, J. (2000). Using "linkage and exchange" to move research into policy at a Canadian foundation. *Health Affairs (Project Hope)*, *19*(3), 236–40. http://dx.doi.org/10.1377/hlthaff.19.3.236 Medline:10812803

Nursing Sector Study Corporation. (2005). *Phase I final report: Building the future: An integrated strategy for nursing human resources in Canada.*

Nursing Sector Study Corporation. (2006). *Phase II final report: Building the future: An integrated strategy for nursing human resources in Canada.*

Nursing Task Force. (1999). *Good nursing, good health: An investment for the 21st century.* Report of the nursing task force.

O'Brien-Pallas, L. (2002). Guest editorial and discourse. Where to from here? *Canadian Journal of Nursing Research*, *33*(4), 3–14. Medline:11998195

O'Brien-Pallas, L. (2003). Leadership in research: About building relationships. *Nursing Leadership (Toronto, Ont.)*, *16*(1), 28–31. Medline:12757300

O'Brien-Pallas, L., Alksnis, C., & Wang, S. (2003a). *Bringing the future into focus: Projecting RN retirement in Canada.* Ottawa, ON: CIHI.

O'Brien-Pallas, L., Alksnis, C., Wang, S., Tomblin Murphy, G., & Meyer, R. (2003b). Trouble on the horizon: Nursing human resources in Ontario, Canada. *International Nursing Perspectives*, *3*(2), 85–94.

O'Brien-Pallas, L., & Baumann, A. (1997). *Health human resources planning in the province of Ontario.* Toronto: Nursing Effectiveness, Utilization and Outcomes Research Unit, University of Toronto and McMaster University.

O'Brien-Pallas, L., & Baumann, A. (2000). Toward evidence-based policy decisions: A case study of nursing health human resources in Ontario, Canada. *Nursing Inquiry*, *7*(4), 248–57. http://dx.doi.org/10.1046/j.1440-1800.2000.00072.x

O'Brien-Pallas, L., Duffield, C., Tomblin Murphy, G., Birch, S., & Meyer, R. (2005). *Nursing workforce planning: Mapping the policy trail.* Geneva, Switzerland: International Council of Nurses.

O'Brien-Pallas, L., Irvine Doran, D., Murray, M., Cockerill, R., Sidani, S., Laurie-Shaw, B., & Lochhaas-Gerlach, J. (2002). Evaluation of a client care delivery model, part 2: Variability in client outcomes in community home nursing. *Nursing Economics*, *20*(1), 13–21, 36. Medline:11892543

O'Brien-Pallas, L., Thomson, D., McGillis Hall, L., Pink, G., Kerr, M., Wang, S., Li, X., & Meyer, R. (2003c). *Evidence based standards for measuring nurse staffing and performance.* Toronto, ON: Nursing Effectiveness, Utilization, and Outcomes Research Unit.

O'Brien-Pallas, L., Tomblin Murphy, G., Baumann, A., & Birch, S. (2001). Framework for analyzing health human resources. In *Future development of information to support the management of nursing resources: Recommendations* (p. 6). Retrieved from https://secure.cihi.ca/free_products/FutureDev.pdf

O'Brien-Pallas, L., Tomblin Murphy, G., Birch, S., Kephart, G., Meyer, R., Eisler, K., ... , & Cook, A. (2007). *Health human resources modelling: Challenging the past, creating the future.* Retrieved from http://www.cfhi-fcass.ca/migrated/pdf/researchreports/ogc/obrien-1_3_25.pdf

O'Brien-Pallas, L., Tomblin Murphy, G., Shamian, J., Li, X.M., Kephart, G., Laschinger, H., ... , & Liu, Y. (2008). *Understanding the costs and outcomes of nurses' turnover in Canadian hospitals (nursing turnover study).* Final report submitted to CIHR.

Sears, K.A. (2009). *The relationship between the nursing work environment and the occurrence of reported paediatric medication administration errors.* Thesis (PhD), University of Toronto, 2009. Retrieved from http://link.library.utoronto.ca/eir/EIRdetail.cfm?Resources__ID=968402&T=F

Simpson, B., Skelton-Green, J., Scott, J.J., & O'Brien-Pallas, L. (2002). Building capacity in nursing: Creating a leadership institute. *Canadian Journal of Nursing Leadership, 15*(3), 22–7. Medline:12395973

Tomblin Murphy, G. (January 2005). *Health human resource planning: An examination of relationships among nursing service utilization, and estimate of population health, and overall health outcomes in the province of Ontario.* Doctoral dissertation.

Tomblin Murphy, G., & O'Brien-Pallas, L. (2002). *How do health human resources policies and practices inhibit change? A plan for the future.* Commission of the future of health care in Canada. Discussion Paper No. 30.

Tomblin Murphy, G., & O'Brien-Pallas, L. (2005). *Guidance document for the development of data sets to support health human resources management in Canada.* Ottawa, ON: CIHI.

World Health Organization. (2002). *Nursing midwifery services: Strategic directions 2002–2008.* Geneva, Switzerland: WHO. Retrieved from http://www.nmh.uts.edu.au/whocc/projects/strategic-directions-2002-2008.pdf

PART THREE

Novel Ways to Structure Learning

While knowledge exchange was a central focus of the CHSRF/CIHR chairs program, developing a new generation of health services researchers who knew how to work in these new relationships was another major objective. In this section, Nancy Edwards uses a research internship developed as part of her chair's program to illustrate the concept of scaling up and its relevant theories. Although originally designed as a program to develop the capacity of researchers in Canada in grantsmanship, linkage, and exchange, the internship has been scaled up in several other countries. Edwards identifies key factors that support scaling up, including features of the internship that were congruent with the characteristics of innovations that diffuse more rapidly, the creation of compatible funding mechanisms, and the influence of temporal dimensions of complex systems change.

In Chapter 8, Ingrid Sketris discusses opportunities and challenges for academic researchers in graduate education and in research on pharmaceutical policy. As was the case with other chairs, her objectives were to: (1) develop capacity in graduate students and junior faculty to conduct research relevant to the needs of decision-makers; (2) conduct research on the ability of policies and programs to provide safe, effective, and affordable drugs; and (3) strengthen links between decision-makers, graduate students, and faculty.

Her particular focus was a key policy challenge: how to provide access to safe, effective, appropriate, and affordable prescription drugs in an environment of new drug technologies, aging populations, rising expenditures, and finite resources. She uses two cases of graduate students conducting service learning to illustrate how these objectives worked in practice. The first involves examining the relinquishment of an older drug technology – wet nebulization respiratory therapy for the treatment of asthma and chronic obstructive lung diseases. The second involves the too-rapid diffusion into blood glucose self-monitoring in patients with type 2 diabetes.

As Alba DiCenso points out in Chapter 9, there has been an important evolution in the nature of the relationship between researchers and decision-makers during the chairs' tenure. While the two groups have tended to work in isolation from each other, early and ongoing involvement of relevant decision-makers in the research process is the best predictor of research use. So highly acknowledged is the importance of this partnership that funders now often require investigators to interact with decision-makers in all phases of their research. As DiCenso makes clear, learning how to engage decision-makers in research is not typically included in traditional research training. She focuses on engaged scholarship as a theoretical framework for the working relationship between researchers and decision-makers. Using the experience of a training program to build capacity in nursing health services research, she describes components of the program designed to prepare researchers to engage with decision-makers. She also outlines a research initiative, led by graduates of the training program, to illustrate social engagement theory, including its benefits, challenges, and lessons learned.

7 Scaling Up for Systems' Changes

NANCY EDWARDS

There are two lively debates underway among health sciences academics that set the stage for this chapter: the first concerns our responsibilities in knowledge translation, and the second concerns our roles in global health. At the heart of both debates is the question of where research, and thus the role of the academic, starts and stops. In this chapter, I consider the intersection of these two debates, as they unfolded in the capacity-building and research activities of my CHSRF/CIHR Nursing Chair in multiple interventions for community health nursing. I use the concept and processes of scaling up as an analytical base to examine my approach. I begin with a brief synopsis of these two central debates and outline the focus of my chair. I then introduce the concept of scaling up and provide a summary of relevant theory. I describe a research internship that was designed as part of my chair and the conditions that supported its international scaling up. I conclude with reflections on pertinent theory to guide scaling-up approaches.

The Role of Academics in Knowledge Translation and Global Health

Academics provide a public good. They are in the business of building research capacity and generating research findings that ultimately may be used for social and health improvement. Achieving excellence in these endeavours paves the way for a strong academic enterprise. An inherently competitive research environment pits academics against one another in the grant submission process and sets the stage for universities to compete for top-notch graduate students, postdoctoral fellows, and research chairs. While these competitive processes and related structural incentives arguably create the conditions that foster research excellence, they can also result in more institution-specific foci that thwart collaborative efforts and encourage academics to think locally rather than broadly. In essence, these structures may discourage scaling up in all facets of academia: education, research, and knowledge translation.

It is pertinent here to ponder whether or not scaling up is an academic tradition. Certainly, the intention to build capacity and to move scientific discovery from bench to product, from emerging concepts to theory, and from insights to services occurs in many aspects of academic life. Thus, scaling up appears to underpin the core academic functions of training and research. However, organizational structures, role-related boundaries, and incentive systems may limit academics' efforts to scale up.

My chair focused on community health nursing, with a particular emphasis on multi-level and multi-strategy programs (Edwards, Mill, & Kothari, 2004). My ten-year vision for the chair included:

- A strong network of community health nursing researchers across Canada who are linked with key decision-makers in government and firmly connected with national and provincial health and nursing associations.
- Timely access of community health nursing managers across Canada to nursing researchers and increased demand for research findings.
- A firmly established mentoring program for community health nursing researchers that supports the development of a strong renewable base of community health nursing researchers.
- Reduced lag time in adopting community health nursing research into practice and curricula.
- Impact of research clearly reflected in design and deployment of multi-component and multi-level community health programs across Canada.

Although the ten-year window for the CHSRF/CIHR chairs program was generous, I was concerned that the usual period required for graduate-level training might seriously curtail opportunities for change if I focused on mentoring doctoral students. This was coupled with the fact that we were just initiating our doctoral program in population health at the University of Ottawa in 2001, and I would not be supervising doctoral students until this program began. Thus, trainees and researchers at various stages of their careers were targeted, including those who were doctoral graduate students, postdoctoral fellows, decision-makers, and junior and senior researchers. A three-month research internship was designed to complement graduate training and provide a means to more rapidly scale up capacity for community health nursing research.

My program of research provided an important training ground for graduate students, postdoctoral fellows, and interns. When I took on my chair award, I was involved in research initiatives in both Canada and China. Several of these initiatives were within programs that had a systems change focus, which provided fertile community laboratories for studies of multi-level and multi-strategy interventions. In this chapter I use, as exemplars, the global health initiatives in which I was involved and in which I became involved during my time as chair.

Scaling Up: Concepts and Theories

Scaling Up

Scaling up is a complex process that has been described in many sectors, including health, engineering, environment, urban planning, business, economics, and international development. Definitions used across sectors are remarkably similar. For example, the International Institute of Rural Reconstruction defines scaling up as "efforts to bring more quality benefits to more people over a wider geographical area more quickly, more equitably and more lastingly" (IIRR, 2000, p. iv). Similarly, in the health sector, Simmon, Fajans, and Ghiron define it as "efforts to increase the impact of innovations successfully tested in pilot or experimental projects so as to benefit more people and to foster policy and program development on a lasting basis" (2008, p. viii). Those who work in poverty reduction describe scaling up as "adapting and expanding positive development experiences in space and time" (China.org, 2004, p. 2).

Successful scale up requires organizational and higher-level system capacities. It is important to distinguish between pilot projects designed as forerunners of scaling up versus those designed for other purposes. Boutique intervention programs are an example of the latter – they are expensive, resource intensive, and tailored to a niche group of participants, and so are not good candidates for scaling up. In contrast, pilot projects that are good candidates are typically characterized by appropriate technology, affordability, and relevance to large segments of the population.

Common to many discussions of scaling-up initiatives are the magnitude, complexity, and intransigence of the problem being addressed (e.g., HIV/AIDS, urban squatter settlements, or the provision of quality education to children in inner city schools) and the urgent need for solutions and a societal response. Analyses of previous failures to adequately scale-up programs have yielded various gaps including: failures to address justice, pro-poor strategies, and governance (Chopra & Ford, 2005; Mehta, 2008); underestimating or ignoring system and absorption capacities in the arenas of health human resource, governance, legal, administrative, and financial systems (Edwards & Roelofs, 2006a; Gillespie, Karklins, Creanga, Khan, & Cho, 2007; Huicho et al., 2005; Hanson, Ranson, Oliveira-Cruz, & Mills, 2003; Nyonator, Awoonor-Williams et al., 2005; World Health Organization, 2008); and making assumptions about system integration that may be relevant now but are fragile or naïve in the long-term (Edwards & Roelofs 2006b; Moreno-Dodson, 2005). Over-emphasizing either horizontal or vertical elements of scaling up has also proven problematic. For instance, the vertical scaling up of anti-retroviral treatments for those living with HIV/AIDS in lower-income countries was planned without due attention to the ways in which it might horizontally distort the delivery of other health services (Koenig, Léandre, & Farmer, 2004; Libamba, Makombe, Harries, Chimzizi, Salaniponi, Schouten et al., 2005). An over-emphasis on the horizontal extension of nurse practitioner roles in Canada created inertia around changes that were required to support this new role at other system levels (i.e., organizational, professionally regulatory, and legislative bodies) (Edwards, Marck, Rowan, & Grinspun, 2011).

These examples suggest the importance of addressing scaling-up processes at an early stage but, as authors in many fields note, scaling up is too often not considered until the post-project phase. Scaling-up strategies that are pertinent to earlier project phases include appraising institutional capacity for scaling up, and developing networks and partnerships that reflect pathways to scaling up from the grassroots to end users (Gündel, Hancock, & Anderson, 2001).

Both temporal and spatial dimensions of scaling up are important. However, the health services literature concentrates on spatiality with a focus on coverage, reach, and accessibility. Indicators to assess these spatial attributes are in common use. The temporal axis for scaling up takes into account the pace of change at each level of the system and the conditions that are required to initiate, sustain, or alter change processes both within and between system levels. Networks and strategic alliances provide a means to build connections horizontally and vertically through a system. They are important strategies for scaling up in studies of training programs, natural resource management, and financing systems (De Souza, 2008; Gallardo, Goldberg, & Randhawa, 2006; IIRR, 2000).

It is important to note that scaling up is not merely another term for concepts like diffusion, spread, and sustainability. Successful scaling-up initiatives involve a systems view, with attention to the characteristics of larger systems needed to support changes that reach those most in need (Edwards & Roelofs, 2006a; Simmons, Fajans, & Ghiron, 2008). Scaling-up approaches must fit the characteristics of what is being introduced, and address both horizontal and vertical system supports.

The Theoretical Base for Scaling Up

The concept of scaling up is rooted in several theories. These theories provide an analytical base for the discussion of a scaling-up example from my chair's program. A précis of these theories and distinctions among them follows.

The first is systems theory (Green, 2006). This theory notes that several processes are critical to scaling up. Throughputs are the mechanisms for change that convert inputs to outcomes. Throughputs that lay the foundation for scaling up operate not only within, but also across, system levels. Thus, if inputs are going to successfully yield multi-level outputs that range, for example, from individual to organizational to regulatory changes, then multi-level mechanisms must be operative. Feedback is a fundamental feature of systems change processes. Feedback mechanisms continuously re-channel outcomes as inputs for the system. These new inputs may be fed into the system level from which they were generated, or into other system levels. The impacts of system change processes occur not only within the system of interest, but also within a larger system of adjacent organizations, sectors, and programs. For instance, secondary outcomes and ripple effects may occur within another system as a consequence of changes in the primary system.

The second pertinent theory comes from the field of innovation diffusion. Rogers' (1995) seminal work continues to provide theoretical grounding for efforts to introduce system innovation. He identifies the characteristics of innovations that enhance their diffusion, and the stages of innovation adoption within a population. He focuses on discrete innovations that are readily described and defined. In his earlier work, for example, Rogers examined the uptake of agricultural innovations such as new seeds and fertilizers. Although Rogers' theory has been applied to innovations that may be considered more complex and less tangible, it is less applicable to innovations that need to be reformed and reshaped across system levels. Thus, innovation diffusion theory provides a stronger base for describing horizontal dissemination processes across the same levels of the system than vertical uptake processes between different ones.

The third and arguably most relevant theory for scaling up is complex adaptation theory (Gunderson & Holling, 2002). The roots of this theory are in ecology. Adaptation uses a whole systems approach that takes into account different levels of and time scales for change. Rather than isolating one particular type of change, adaptation theory reflects many concurrent change processes both within and between system levels. Thus, it considers the many converging contexts for change and helps describe the conditions for antagonistic and complimentary effects. This theory also identities factors, such as connectedness and social capital, that influence scaling up between vertical system levels. In contrast, factors that produce inter-system rigidity include autocratic governance structures and historically oppressive power hierarchies.

Given the nature of scaling up, all three theories can help to explain what comprises a complex set of change processes. In summary, systems theory provides insights on how inputs are converted to outputs and how these in turn are channelled into the system through critical feedback processes. Innovation diffusion theory notes that the characteristics of both what is being diffused and how it is diffused influence the uptake of innovations. Complex adaptation theory describes how context influences dynamic changes between micro, meso, and macro system levels. Complex adaptation theory also explains how change processes interact across varying time scales at different system levels, with sustainable change at one system level potentially reinforced or undermined by change processes at other levels.

Creating the Conditions for Scaling Up

Requirements of the CHSRF/CIHR chairs program pushed applicants to "think outside the box" and develop novel structures and approaches to work with trainees and carry out knowledge exchange activities on a national scale. In outlining a vision for our proposed programs, we had to describe how we would enhance applied research capacity and improve linkage and exchange within the health system. The push to think provincially and nationally rather than just locally was perhaps a more implicit than explicit interpretation of the award requirements. The competition was national in scope and several of the chairs had a very specific focus. Thus, it seemed implausible that the review committee would be satisfied with an application describing a program concentrated in a single university. We had to provide a ten-year vision for the chair, and the criterion used to assign a top-level rating for this vision was "the main thrust of the proposal is so directly significant that it will be of compelling interest to managers or policy makers through the next ten years." The duration of the chairs program encouraged applicants to consider what significant shifts we might effect in our fields of research over a decade. The chairs program's dual emphasis on capacity building and strategic links with health system actors on one hand and its focus on mentorship on the other encouraged applicants to carefully consider the potential forums for interaction they might create for trainees and decision-makers. The program explicitly expected us to provide evidence of formalized links with decision-makers and encouraged us to describe how our research program might become a resource for the country rather than just our university. Finally, we had to provide a substantial amount of documentation detailing the explicit support for our respective programs from those in key positions in our universities and in the decision-making settings linked to our programs of research. This helped to ensure that the long-term commitments we would need to realize our goals would not be threatened by a change in local leadership.

These application requirements set the stage for thinking about ways to scale up our work. The thrust of the CHSRF/CIHR chairs program threw the more typical university-centric approach off-kilter right from the start. The chairs were asked to conceptualize their award as national in scope and reach. While each chair was necessarily housed within an academic institution and had to demonstrate that it supported their proposed work, the chairs program intended to make the chairs' work nationally accessible. Thus, the primary beneficiaries of the program were to exist beyond the trainees and decision-makers who might participate in local training programs and individual institutions. In the next section, I describe how the design of a research internship addressed these specifications and link the internship to the international elements of my research program.

Research Internship Design

The design of a research internship was an integral part of my program. I initially conceived the internship as a three-month on-site program intended to complement graduate training and help fast-track nurses' research careers by improving their ability to write research grant proposals, publish and translate knowledge, and collaborate with interdisciplinary teams (Smith & Edwards, 2003; Edwards & MacDonald, 2009). Those selected for the internship had at least a master's degree. The internship was one of several training components, and from the outset I envisioned the involvement of other trainees in the internship program. I planned to offer the internship for three or four years and prepare a cohort of twenty nurses in Canada. The internship was one of several strategies I used to build a national network of community health nurse researchers.

My chair award financially supported the first group of six interns. News of the internship spread, in part through a series of site visits I made to various universities and colleges across the country. Several nursing deans and directors expressed interest in the program and committed funds to send faculty members. The structure of the program evolved considerably – it began entirely on site, but grew to include a combination of on-site and distance learning activities. By the sixth year of my chair, one hundred interns from nine Canadian provinces had participated, as had fourteen postdoctoral fellows whom I had supervised during the same period. Participants came from universities, health service delivery organizations, and professional nursing associations. Approximately 50 per cent had a master's degree while the other half either had a PhD or were enrolled in a PhD program.

Reaching out to colleagues across the country engaged some nurses who would not typically have been attracted to research training opportunities. The internship was designed to increase accessibility. For example, distance education was conducted via audio, rather than video, teleconference, as the costs and accessibility of the latter were prohibitive for some institutions.

Setting the Stage for an International Internship

Though the potential for an international arm of the internship was present at the outset of my chair, it only began to take hold in the fourth year. When I took on the chair, I was the Canadian director for a development project in China. This bilateral initiative was funded by the Canadian International Development Agency (CIDA) and undertaken in partnership with the maternal and child health division of the Yunnan Ministry of Health. Yunnan is a province of 44 million people, situated in southwest China. In brief, the six-year project involved the use of participatory training and management and evaluation strategies to tackle high rates of maternal, infant, and child mortality (Edwards & Roelofs, 2005). Our work targeted ten poor counties where the residents were predominantly ethnic minorities and subsistence farmers. Although CHSRF agreed that I could continue this work during the tenure of my chair award, it subsequently raised a number of concerns about the relevance of this international project to my chair.

These concerns came to a head when CIDA asked me to lead a team that would examine the potential to extend this participatory project to three western provinces in China and design a development program for implementation. In essence, CIDA wanted to scale up the initiative to other parts of China that were also very poor and where maternal and child health concerns were paramount. The pertinence of these health issues and the lack of similarities between the Canadian and the Chinese healthcare systems led CHSRF to question the relevance of this work to my chair. At the same time, my dean questioned my involvement in the new project, as it appeared to concentrate more heavily on development and training than on research. I argued forcefully for my involvement in this initiative with both CHSRF and my dean.

From my perspective, the new initiative in China would provide another community laboratory to further examine multilevel and multistrategy systems change. Although at the time, the policies of CIDA did not permit my team to explicitly include a major research thrust within a development aid project, there were many opportunities to undertake operational research and offer training. I was given the go-ahead to proceed with the initiative in Western China. Ultimately, for a variety of reasons, CIDA and the Chinese government did not approve the new initiative for funding. However, through this process, I had made the case for the relevance of international development work to my chair and had developed a better understanding of the political conditions required for a major scaling-up initiative. In part, this set the stage for expanding the research internship to an international scale.

Several circumstances converged to prompt formal internationalization of the research internship. A former postdoctoral fellow, then working with the Office of Nursing Policy, Health Canada, met colleagues from Jamaica and Barbados during an invitational workshop to discuss a plan for managed migration for the Caribbean. She mentioned the internship, and colleagues from the University of West Indies, who had recently established the first master's program for nurses in the Caribbean and were converting many of their undergraduate courses for distance delivery in the region, expressed their interest. Also at this invitational workshop was a senior academic who had previously held the role as director of our school and dean of our faculty. She was invited to spend a week at the University of West Indies, Jamaica, to provide research mentorship. Finally, I had been involved in international development initiatives for many years, and had a personal interest in the potential to extend the research internship to lower income countries.

In the meantime, several individuals with extensive international networks from the Canadian Nurses Association and other Canadian universities had completed the internship and identified its potential as an international training resource for nurses in lower income countries. My relationships with a number of national decision-makers had been considerably strengthened through their participation in the internship as guest speakers; as external reviewers for, and co-applicants on, research projects; and as mentors for postdoctoral fellows. These decision-makers and their respective organizations started to emerge as nodes within a network. In discussions with one of the senior decision-makers, we explored the possibility of supporting an international intern from Jamaica to join a portion of the program. A pilot initiative, funded by the Office of Nursing Policy, began and allowed us to gauge the relevance of the internship model and its curriculum for international partners. In the subsequent year, we again applied for funding from the Office of Nursing Policy. We selected evidence-based practice as a focus, and two more colleagues from Jamaica completed the internship. I subsequently visited Jamaica and Barbados and made connections with national and regional nursing associations, chief nursing officers, directors of nursing departments, and the Pan American Health Organization.

Working with the Canadian Nurses Association, and in an effort to better understand the research capacity training needs and constraints of colleagues in lower income countries, we conducted interviews with national nursing stakeholders in nine countries (Edwards, Webber, Mill, Kahwa, & Roelofs, 2009). We then held an invitational workshop with representatives from several national associations in Canada, including CHSRF. We asked participants to reflect on the insights offered by international partners. They concluded that there was strong support for an international version of the internship.

An international research platform for such a program was essential. By this stage, both the development projects and a funded research project in China were drawing to a close. However, my interest in international research had not waned. In the fifth year of the internship, I prepared a research project that focused on how nurses' involvement in policy shaped programs targeting HIV and AIDS. Several interns (including colleagues from the Canadian Nurses Association) and postdoctoral fellows joined as co-investigators. We wrote a grant proposal for submission to the Canadian Institutes of Health Research that was (overly) ambitious, (too) expensive, and involved working with (too many) nursing partners in seven countries and four regions (Sub-Saharan Africa, Caribbean, Latin America, and Southeast Asia). Although this project was not funded, it allowed us to work together as a research team and identify a critical area of interest that we wanted to pursue. The experience also led us to rethink how geographically expansive the project should be.

The final element that set the stage for internationalizing the internship was a funding opportunity from the Canadian Global Health Research Initiative. The initiative called for proposals that integrated capacity building and research. We merged our plans to expand the internship internationally with our interest in researching the role of nurses in policy for HIV and AIDS. We subsequently obtained funding for a program of research entitled "Strengthening Nurses' Capacity in HIV Policy Development in Sub-Saharan Africa and the Caribbean" (Edwards, Kahwa, Kaseje, Mill, Webber, & Roelofs, 2007). I led this project, along with a physician colleague from Kenya and the nursing colleague from Jamaica who had completed the internship in 2005. Three African nations and one Caribbean country (all Commonwealth nations) participated. The internship was a major capacity-building component of this program of research.

The Internationalized Internship

The inaugural internationalized internship was held in Canada in 2008, with interns participating from all countries that are involved in our HIV and AIDS program of research. In 2009, the internship was held at Great Lakes University of Kisumu, Kenya, followed by Jamaica in 2010 and South Africa in 2011. It was repeated in Kenya in 2012.

Many core elements of the original internship program were retained but adapted to the realities of a weak communications infrastructure, uneven Internet access, and strained nursing human resources in participating lower- and middle-income countries. We scaled up the internship, not only to build the interns' research skills, but also to focus on reaching other nurses, decision-making partners, and research systems in the countries where the interns worked.

As part of the internationalization process, a wider range of speakers participated in the internship, with the involvement of senior researchers, research funding agencies, and decision-makers from Africa and the Caribbean. For example, chief nursing officers from Canada, Kenya, and Jamaica jointly participated, via an audio teleconference, on a panel to discuss their roles and provide suggestions on how nurse researchers might work with government partners in their respective countries. In addition, interns met with senior scientists in the Kenyan Medical Research Institute during the on-site portion in Kisumu, where they had a chance to discuss the importance of and opportunities for nurses' involvement in research. These learning strategies allowed interns to build their confidence in discussing research ideas with senior decision-makers and to extend their networks with these individuals.

At the same time, these strategies created a forum in which to engage senior scientists and decision-makers in discussions about nurses' involvement in research. Beneath this approach is an effort to scale up opportunities for nurses' involvement in research, not only as data collectors as is traditionally the case (Edwards, Webber, Mill, Kahwa, & Roelofs, 2009), but also as investigators. Thus, scaling up the internship allowed us to reach other system levels in other countries. It also created opportunities for discussions about how more biomedically oriented research systems can be adjusted to support nurse-led research. For instance, during the Jamaican internship, senior university officials discussed the structures needed to support nursing research in the region. Since interns were encouraged to consider how they could take what they learned from their conversations with decision-makers and research funding agencies staff back to their own settings, these types of discussions were replicated following the internship.

As described above, the internship was coupled with our funded research program on HIV and AIDS. Some of the interns were directly involved in that program as co-investigators, collaborators, or research assistants, while others were members of either national advisory committees or leadership hubs established as part of the program. Some interns had no a priori connection to the program but became familiar with it during the internship, since it was used as a basis for training on topics such as qualitative analysis, mixed methods study designs, governance structures for international research projects, and engaging decision-makers in research studies. Following completion of the internship, all interns who had been sponsored with funding from the research program were required to share what they had learned through training initiatives in their own countries. Such initiatives included skill-building workshops for leadership hubs related to the policy-making process and seminars for research assistants on using qualitative software and conducting qualitative data analysis. In this way, the interns' newly developed skill sets were immediately transferable, with receptor nodes for the introduction of these skills having been pre-established within the program of research. These activities were intended to make the learning gained during the internship accessible to others, consistent with the equity goals of scaling up.

Furthermore, since the aim of the leadership hubs was to consider research findings that emerged from the study and develop action plans within their own district to address HIV and AIDS, and since each country had a national advisory committee that linked district research efforts to provincial and national policy and program initiatives, interns' involvement in this platform of research provided them with links through all system levels of decision-making. The engagement of interns with the leadership hubs and national advisory committees provided a vehicle to enhance inter-system fluidity for the flow of research ideas.

New initiatives were developed to support institutional change within each of the participating countries. For example, in 2008, interns and postdoctoral fellows developed a research project to examine infrastructure supports for research by nurses in each of the partner countries. During the 2009 internship, some trainees joined an initiative that aimed to improve reciprocal, virtual exchanges for community health clinical placements among participating countries, while others began work on a project to examine the role of nurses in research associations within their respective countries.

Lessons Learned

It is premature to determine how successful our international scaling-up efforts have been. Many new challenges await us as we work with nursing colleagues in lower-and middle-income countries – colleagues who directly experience the many repercussions of an acute scarcity of health human resources. However, we did learn lessons about the types of supports required for academics to scale up initiatives focused on building research capacity. Several interrelated features of the internship and areas of activity helped create conditions for scaling up the internship. These include characteristics of the internship that are compatible with innovation diffusion, the creation of funding mechanisms to support this type of work, and attending to the temporal dimensions of complex systems change.

Characteristics of the Internship

The internship was an innovation. Several of its characteristics were consistent with features of innovation that Rogers describes as enhancing diffusion. These included its relative advantage, compatibility, observability, and trialability (Rogers, 1995). The relative advantage of an innovation has to do with its perceived advantages over usual practices. Compatibility concerns the fit between the innovation and the usual behaviour of those who are targeted to take up the innovation. An innovation with high observability can readily be seen or experienced by others who have not yet taken it up. Trialability pertains to the possibility of trying out the innovation before deciding whether or not to adopt it.

The internship was perceived as having relative advantage over the more common model of expecting academic nurses to find their way onto research teams, develop a program of research, and submit high-quality research proposals when they often had no formal training in writing research grant proposals or working on research initiatives with decision-makers. The internship provided a means to fast-track learning in these essential skills. Academic leaders in Canada, and now internationally, have been keen to encourage recently minted doctoral graduates and junior faculty to attend it.

The internship was compatible with the requirements of academics for scholarly productivity and with increasing expectations from funding agencies that health systems researchers work closely with decision-makers. Learners were able to pick and choose activities in line with these requirements and expectations, and could select from shorter- or longer-term options. For example, in addition to their own research project, in which decision-makers were encouraged to be involved, interns had to join at least one additional project team with a focus on proposal development, data analysis, knowledge translation, or manuscript preparation.

The repeated annual offerings of the internship allowed other colleagues to observe the program before deciding whether or not to try it. We attempted to enhance observability by inviting the interns' home colleagues to join selected internship sessions. Decision-makers' engagement in various internship activities also increased the program's observability. For instance, we obtained permission for all the interns to join events organized by Health Canada's Office of Nursing Policy during nurses' week, and we received an invitation for all interns to participate in a health forum that was held at the Canadian Nurses Association and involved their senior staff. In Kenya, nursing leaders from three national organizations shared perspectives on research capacity and national priorities with interns, and then acted as discussants when interns identified potential research initiatives that might be pertinent to the leaders' identified priorities. These types of fora led some decision-making partners to encourage their staff to apply for the internship.

Trialability was introduced by providing the school of nursing at the University of West Indies with an opportunity to send several colleagues to the internship. Their feedback on the suitability of the internship for lower- and middle-income countries helped us adjust the internship model. We also asked stakeholders from a variety of international settings to provide input on the compatibility of the internship within their context. We were concerned that the requirements of a graduate degree and the length of the internship might not be realistic given health human resource constraints in lower income countries. On their advice, we maintained the requirement of a graduate degree and initially shortened the length of the internship from 2.5 months to 1.5 months and then to one month, although we increased the period of full-time commitment.

Compatible Funding Mechanisms

The objectives and learning approaches of the internship were aimed at researchers in traditional academic settings and decision-makers in health service institutions, professional associations, and government organizations. This was in keeping with one of the foci of the CHSRF/CIHR chairs program, which was to stimulate interactions between researchers and decision-makers. Thus, the initial funding mechanism created for the chairs program set the stage for scaling up the internship within Canada. Subsequently, the joint efforts of university researchers and those in key decision-making positions enabled us to internationalize the internship.

CHSRF helped create the conditions for scaling up innovations undertaken by the chair in other ways. The ten-year duration of the chair, and the explicit requirement of university leaders' support for its activities, provided an opportunity to incubate novel capacity-building initiatives that fell outside the usual types of training programs funded by universities. Furthermore, CHSRF itself set out to scale up its approaches, notably within CIHR, thereby providing the funding mechanism that ultimately supported the international scale up of the internship. Specifically, CHSRF worked to transfer innovations it had successfully launched to CIHR. Among these innovations were the introduction of merit review panels for health services research, with both researchers and decision-makers providing peer review; the design of the chairs program, which included a strong focus on mentorship, linkage, and exchange; and the development of knowledge translation tools and strategies such as the knowledge use assessment tool (Kothari, Edwards, Hamel, & Judd, 2009). Subsequently, CHSRF transferred some of these innovations to joint funding initiatives in which CIHR was involved. For example, four agencies, including CIHR (but not CHSRF), formed the Global Health Research Initiative and called for funding international research programs that incorporated specific requirements for mentorship, capacity-building, and knowledge translation strategies. This was the call for funds that our team successfully responded to for the HIV and AIDS research program.

Temporal Dimensions of Complex Systems Change

Although it may have been possible to scale up the internship internationally earlier, many conditions needed to be put in place for growth to begin. The temporal aspects of scaling up are important and in this case involved: (1) building a strategic alliance between researchers and the Canadian Nurses Association, which has a long, ongoing history of working successfully with nursing associations in many countries; (2) establishing a cohort of intern graduates and a scaffold of trainees at various stages of their research careers; (3) developing momentum for an international internship and permission for it, both from the funding agency for the chair and from the university of the chair holder; and (4) obtaining funding for a large-scale, international research platform that could help support the internship.

A complex set of relationships, activities, and networks were essential for scaling up. An international team of individuals who became an informal network during the period of the chair enabled these efforts. Through a shared vision and complementary leadership roles, we were able to leverage the strengths of our respective institutions in academic, professional, and governmental arenas to scale up the internship. In the section below, I return to the theories for scaling up and consider their utility using the internship example.

Scaling-Up Theories Revisited

Important links between two systems of innovation ultimately converged to create the conditions necessary for scaling up the internship from national to international levels. Specifically, the internship for training community health researchers that I developed and the research funding system directly influenced by CHSRF jointly enabled this scale up.

Consistent with innovation diffusion theory, we tested a potential international prototype of the internship with international colleagues from Jamaica, and subsequently adapted it. This model was observable by senior colleagues from both nursing organizations in Canada and Jamaica, who participated in the internship as speakers, interns, or postdoctoral fellows. The internship itself had to have demonstrated potential for international partners, and my university had to support its international focus. The dean of my faculty was involved as a speaker in the Jamaican institution from which we initially invited interns, which helped to forge system links that we continue to build. In addition, existing partnerships with the Great Lakes University of Kisumu and with a teaching hospital in Kampala, Uganda, were the basis for developing our multi-partnered program of research on HIV and AIDS, which included the internship.

The pertinence of complex adaptation theory played out a number of times. In 2009, our team was asked to present our HIV and AIDS project to the United Nations Commission on the Status of Women. The International Development Research Centre also invited a colleague from the University of Western Cape, South Africa, to present on the same panel. A series of meetings followed, and we briefly discussed the potential for the internship to be offered in South Africa. In the meantime, in a seemingly unrelated set of events, the Atlantic Philanthropic Organization had run a competition to build nursing research capacity in South Africa. In meetings, the leaders of two schools of nursing in South Africa that received this funding indicated they would like to use the internship as one means to strengthen scholarship. Plans for running the internship at Northwest University were subsequently developed.

Although these events appear serendipitous, complex adaptation theory suggests otherwise. The overall direction of change that underlies their convergence is a groundswell of effort to strengthen nurses' engagement in research and scholarship. Calls for this change have been ongoing for several decades (Edwards, Webber, Mill, Kahwa, & Roelofs, 2009). The health human resources crisis, the debate on task-shifting and the profession of nursing, and calls for interdisciplinary approaches in science and research have all created the dynamics for change that supported scaling up the internship. Many initiatives will be required to introduce sustainable improvements in nurses' capacity to lead research and use it for systems change. However, the internship's perceived relevance for upcoming nurse scholars, its timeliness given the impending health human resources crisis, and its adaptability to participants from different political, geographic, and research intensive contexts all created the conditions necessary for its successful scale up.

Conclusion

CHSRF's initial requirements for the chairs helped to set the conditions required for scaling up an innovative research internship. Initial plans were to offer the internship only within Canada. However, a network of international colleagues who shared a common set of principles regarding the contribution of academics to global health provided the impetus for scaling up the research internship internationally.

Theories of innovation diffusion, systems change, and complex adaptation underlie successful scale-up approaches. The application of these theories to the internship illustrates that innovation within the internship itself, temporal conditions that acted collaboratively over time, and feedback processes that demonstrated the outcomes and impact of the internship all contributed to its successful scale up.

REFERENCES

China.org. (2004). Global learning process for scaling up poverty reduction and conference in Shanghai, May 25–7, 2004. Retrieved 29 July 2009 from http://www.china.org.cn/english/MATERIAL/90993.htm

Chopra, M., & Ford, N. (2005). Scaling up health promotion interventions in the era of HIV/AIDS: Challenges for a rights based approach. *Health Promotion International, 20*(4), 383–90. http://dx.doi.org/10.1093/heapro/dai018 Medline:16061497

De Souza, R-M. (2008). Scaling up integrated population, health and environment approaches in the Philippines: A review of early experiences. Washington, DC: World Wildlife Fund and the Population Reference Bureau. Retrieved 4 August 2009 from http://worldwildlife.org/publications/scaling-up-integrated-population-health-and-environment-approaches-in-the-philippines-a-review-of-early-experiences

Edwards, N., Marck, P., Rowan, M., & Grinspun, D. (2011). Understanding whole systems change in health care: The case of nurse practitioners in Canada. *Policy, Politics & Nursing Practice, 12*(1), 4–17. http://dx.doi.org/10.1177/1527154411403816 Medline:21555317

Edwards, N., & Roelofs, S. (2005). Participatory approaches in the co-design of a comprehensive referral system. *L'Infirmiere Canadienne, 6*(8), 13–16.

Edwards, N., & Roelofs, S. (2006a). Developing management systems with cross-cultural fit: Assessing international differences in operational systems. *The International Journal of Health Planning and Management, 21*(1), 55–73. http://dx.doi.org/10.1002/hpm.825 Medline:16604849

Edwards, N.C., & Roelofs, S.M. (2006b). Sustainability: The elusive dimension of international health projects. *Canadian Journal of Public Health, 97*(1), 45–9. Medline:16512328

Edwards, N., Kahwa, E., Kaseje, D., Mill, J., Webber, J., & Roelofs, S. (2007). Strengthening health care systems for HIV and AIDS in sub-Saharan Africa and the Caribbean: A program of research. *Caribbean Journal of Nursing and Midwifery, 2*, 29–36.

Edwards, N., & MacDonald, J.A. (2009). Building nurses' capacity in community health services. *International Journal of Nursing Education Scholarship, 6*(1), e25. http://dx.doi.org/10.2202/1548-923X.1760 Medline:19725806

Edwards, N., Webber, J., Mill, J., Kahwa, E., & Roelofs, S. (2009). Building capacity for nurse-led research. *International Nursing Review, 56*(1), 88–94. http://dx.doi.org/10.1111/j.1466-7657.2008.00683.x Medline:19239521

Edwards, N., Mill, J., & Kothari, A.R. (2004). Multiple intervention research programs in community health. *The Canadian Journal of Nursing Research, 36*(1), 40–54. Medline:15133918

Gallardo, J., Goldberg, M., & Randhawa, B. (2006). Strategic alliances to scale up financial services in rural areas. World Bank working paper #76. Washington, DC: World Bank. Retrieved 4 August 2009 from http://www.icba.coop/images/stories/pdf/strategicalliances.pdf

Gillespie, D., Karklins, S., Creanga, A., Khan, S., & Cho, N. (2007). Scaling up health technologies report. Retrieved 4 August 2009 from http://www.jhsph.edu/research/centers-and-institutes/bill-and-melinda-gates-institute-for-population-and-reproductive-health/_pdf/publications/scalingup_report.pdf

Gündel, S., Hancock, J., & Anderson, S. (2001). Scaling-up strategies for research in natural resources management: A comparative review. Retrieved 29 July 2009, from http://www.nrsp.org.uk/database/documents/195.pdf

Green, L.W. (2006). Public health asks of systems science: To advance our evidence-based practice, can you help us get more practice-based evidence? *American Journal of Public Health, 96*(3), 406–9. http://dx.doi.org/10.2105/AJPH.2005.066035 Medline:16449580

Gunderson, L.H., & Holling, C.S. (2002). *Panarchy: Understanding transformations in human and natural systems*. Washington, DC: Island Press.

Hanson, K., Ranson, M.K., Oliveira-Cruz, V., & Mills, A. (2003). Expanding access to priority health interventions: A framework for understanding the constraints to scaling up. *Journal of Knowledge Management, 15*, 1–14.

Huicho, L., Dávila, M., Campos, M., Drasbek, C., Bryce, J., & Victoria, C.G. (2005). Scaling up integrated management of childhood illness to the national level: Achievements and challenges in Peru. *Health Policy and Planning, 20*(1), 14–24. http://dx.doi.org/10.1093/heapol/czi002 Medline:15689426

IIRR. (2000). Going to scale: Can we bring more benefits to more people more quickly? Silang, Philippines: International Institute of Rural Reconstruction.

Kothari, A., Edwards, N., Hamel, N., & Judd, M. (2009). Is research working for you? Validating a tool to examine the capacity of health organizations to use research. *Implementation Science: IS*, 4(46), 1–9. http://dx.doi.org/10.1186/1748-5908-4-46 Medline:19627601

Koenig, S.P., Léandre, F., & Farmer, P.E. (2004). Scaling-up HIV treatment programmes in resource-limited settings: The rural Haiti experience. *AIDS (London, England)*, *18*(Suppl 3), S21–5. http://dx.doi.org/10.1097/00002030-200406003-00005 Medline:15322480

Libamba, E., Makombe, S., Harries, A.D., Chimzizi, R., Salaniponi, F.M., Schouten, E.J., & Mpazanje, R. (2005). Scaling up antiretroviral therapy in Africa: Learning from tuberculosis control programmes – the case of Malawi. *International Journal of Tuberculosis and Lung Disease*, *9*(10), 1062–71. Medline:16229216

Mehta, M. (2008). Assessing microfinance for water and sanitation: Exploring opportunities for sustainable scaling up. Retrieved 31 July 2009 from http://www.gatesfoundation.org/learning/Documents/assessing-microfinance-wsh-2008.pdf.

Moreno-Dodson, B. (Ed.). (2005). *Reducing poverty on a global scale: Learning and innovation for development: Findings from the Shanghai global learning initiative.* Washington, DC: World Bank.

Nyonator, F.K., Awoonor-Williams, J.K., Phillips, J.F., Jones, T.C., & Miller, R.A. (2005). The Ghana community-based health planning and services initiative for scaling up service delivery innovation. *Health Policy and Planning*, *20*(1), 25–34. http://dx.doi.org/10.1093/heapol/czi003 Medline:15689427

Rogers, E.M. (1995). *Diffusion of innovations* (4th ed.). New York: Free Press.

Simmons, R., Fajan, P., & Ghiron, L. (2008). *Scaling up health service delivery.* Geneva, Switzerland: WHO Press.

Smith, D., & Edwards, N. (2003). Innovation. Building research capacity. *The Canadian Nurse*, *99*(9), 23–7. Medline:14621530

World Health Organization. (2008). Towards universal access: Scaling up priority HIV/AIDS interventions in the health sector. Retrieved 29 July 2009 from http://www.who.int/hiv/pub/2009progressreport/en

8 Service Learning within a Multi-Stakeholder Pharmaceutical Program and Policy Arena

INGRID S. SKETRIS

In this chapter, I describe a Dalhousie University academic graduate-level service learning program, the Drug Use Management and Policy Residency Program, and its impact. I discuss the opportunities and challenges I faced in applying the service learning model to the study of pharmaceutical policy. I use case studies to illustrate the model, and show that scientific evidence produced by academic researchers and their graduate trainees can help inform the health system's pharmaceutical programs and policies, physicians' prescribing, and patients' drug use.

There are over 16,000 marketed therapeutic drug products for humans available in Canada (A. Karaokcu, personal communications, 2 September 2009). Over $25 billion a year is spent on prescription drugs in the community: public drug insurance programs pay 45 per cent, private insurance companies pay 37 per cent, and patients pay 18 per cent (Canadian Institute for Health Information, 2009). Another $1.5 billion is spent on drugs used in hospital (Canadian Institute for Health Information, 2006). In addition, pharmaceutical companies promote their drugs with one representative for every eleven physicians and an estimated budget of $500 million annually for meetings with healthcare professionals (Kondro, 2007). While drugs have a major role in preventing and treating disease and ameliorating quality of life, they also cause drug-related morbidity (Zed et al., 2008). To provide patients with access to drugs, Canada has a suite of pharmaceutical programs administered by the federal and provincial/territorial governments. It does not have a national comprehensive drug use system to determine if the drugs individual patients receive are safe, effective, and affordable, although parts of such a system are in place (Sketris, Langille Ingram, & Lummis, 2007).

The program my Dalhousie colleagues and I developed uses service learning and knowledge transfer concepts. Service learning is a type of experiential learning. A service learning approach brings students' knowledge and skills to contribute to solving real problems decision-makers face (ASPH Council of Public Health Practice Coordinators, 2004; Stanton, Giles, & Cruz, 1999). In my program, graduate trainees develop policy-relevant evidence by conducting a literature synthesis or research project in line with the CHSRF/CIHR linkage and exchange method and using principles from knowledge transfer (Lomas, 2000a, 2000b; Graham & Tetroe, 2007, 2009; Lavis et al., 2003a; Landry, Amara, Pablos-Mendes, Shademani, & Gold, 2006; Greenhalgh et al., 2004; Jacobson, Butterill, & Goering, 2003).

Background

In 2000, I received an education, research, and linkage chair funded by CHSRF/CIHR and cosponsored by the Nova Scotia Health Research Foundation (NSHRF). As a chair holder, I focused on a key policy challenge: how to provide access to safe, effective, appropriate, and affordable prescription drugs. My research studies the use of pharmaceuticals after they are marketed and evaluates management strategies and policies that influence drug use. Along with a principal academic appointment in pharmacy, I have held appointments in health services administration, computer science, nursing, and community health and epidemiology. The specific objectives of my chair's program are:

1) To develop capacity in graduate students and junior faculty to conduct research relevant to the needs of decision-makers who manage pharmaceutical programs in primary care, continuing care, acute care institutions, or provincial governments;
2) To research the effectiveness of policies and programs to provide safe, effective, and affordable drugs;
3) To strengthen links between decision-makers, graduate students, and academic researchers.

My chair's program has an advisory committee composed of representatives from Dalhousie University's administration, faculty, and students; the Nova Scotia provincial department of health; and the local and national healthcare community. The mandate of this advisory committee is to provide monitoring and advice regarding the chair's strategic plan, a wide range of expertise and stakeholder input on programs, and policy advice on request. The committee also helps promote the program (Sketris, 2007b). The chair's program has evolved over time with the guidance of the advisory committee, which encouraged me to plan strategically in the first year of my chair in order to engage government and health system decision-makers, academic colleagues, and trainees in the process to determine strategic programs and specific projects to undertake and tactics to use. One of the key strategic components we identified was the Drug Use Management and Policy Residency Program. To create this program, we received assistance from a policy analyst seconded from the provincial government who helped identify the potential partners in the Nova Scotia pharmaceutical policy community and relevant decision-makers for our knowledge transfer activities. In addition, in 2003, the residency program coordinator attended a service learning course offered by the Community-Campus Partnerships for Health (CCPH) at its third annual Advanced Service-Learning Institute in San Jose, California. The Drug Use Management and Policy Research Residency Program was later featured on the CCPH website (Community-Campus Partnerships for Health, 2004). My colleagues and I implemented the principles from the course to a graduate training experience (Conrad, Murphy, & Sketris, 2005).

The Drug Policy Environment

In order to understand the external environment in which we conduct research and place our students, I begin by describing the pharmaceutical policy community in Nova Scotia and some of the challenges related to drug policy. (See Box 8.1 for a brief overview of the broader Canadian pharmaceutical policy context that influences that in Nova Scotia.) I also describe the organizations I work with in Nova Scotia and their key roles.

BOX 8.1 THE CANADIAN DRUG POLICY CONTEXT: THE ROLE OF THE FEDERAL GOVERNMENT

The federal government sets the legislative framework for drug control; approves drugs and monitors their safety, effectiveness, and quality; determines the maximum prices for patented medicines; participated in the National Pharmaceuticals Strategy and provides some funding towards a program run by the Canadian Agency for Drugs and Technologies in Health to evaluate the clinical and cost effectiveness of drugs; and funds and manages drug programs for specific groups (e.g., registered First Nations, Inuit, recognized Innu people, federal employees, the military, veterans meeting eligibility criteria, certain incarcerated individuals, and the Royal Canadian Mounted Police) among other functions (Health Canada, 2008; Metge & Sketris, 2007, Tierney et al., 2008, Paris & Docteur, 2007).

A particular feature of the Canadian healthcare system is that the Canada Health Act only requires provincial governments to pay for drugs administered in hospitals (Applied Management & Fraser Group Trisat Resources, 2002; Freund et al., 2000; Lindsey & West, 1999; Romanow, 2002). The Canada Health Act does not mandate provincial nonhospital (pharmacare) programs. Each province has the discretion to develop its own pharmacare, and so coverage varies widely, as does the approach to subsidizing and monitoring the delivery of pharmaceuticals for patients in hospitals, long-term care, and home care. While the approaches to pharmacare programs funded by the federal and provincial governments differ, the objectives are similar and include providing access to necessary drug therapy, limiting access to ineffective or unsafe therapy, responding to patient's concerns and preferences, treating patients equitably, and delivering programs efficiently. Some provinces provide some level of coverage for all residents while other provinces provide coverage only for select groups such as seniors and low-income recipients. Pharmacare programs also employ a variety of patient cost sharing mechanisms (Metge & Sketris, 2007; Freund et al., 2000; Lindsey & West, 1999; Bacovsky, 1997; Applied Management & Fraser Group Trisat Resources, 2002; Lexchin, 1996; Grégoire et al., 2001).

Figure 8.1 The Pharmaceutical Policy Community in Nova Scotia

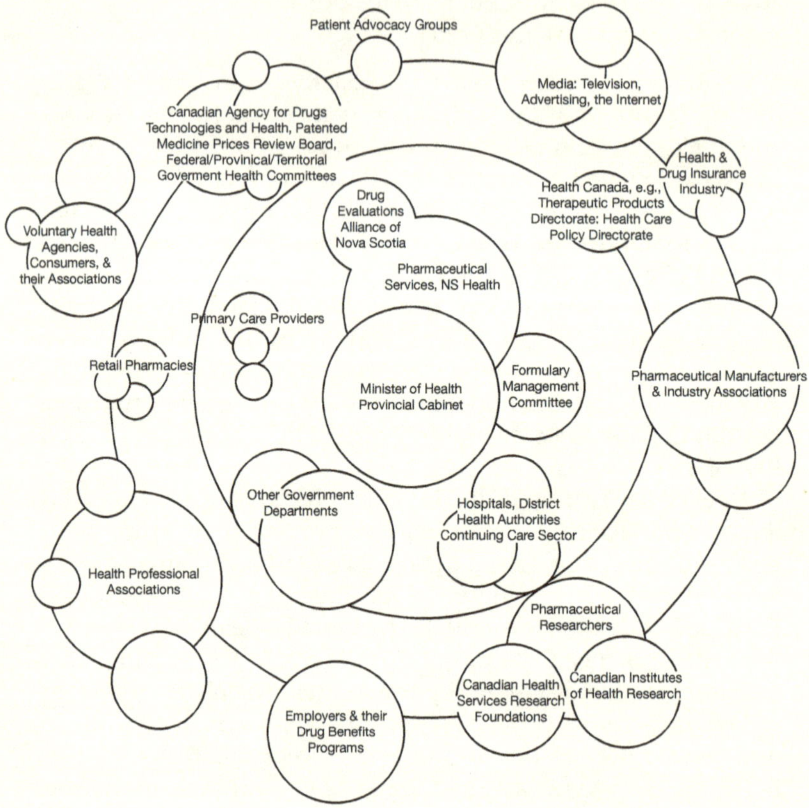

Canadian provinces and territories play a large role in delivery of pharmaceutical programs within the federal government's frameworks (Metge & Sketris, 2007; Paris & Docteur, 2007). Figure 8.1 provides a picture of the pharmaceutical policy community in Nova Scotia. The position of an actor in this figure represents its involvement and influence on provincial drug policy. Those at the centre of the figure exert a more direct and immediate influence on drug policy. The pharmaceutical services division of the Department of Health briefs the minister of health with evidence-based information provided by the Drug Evaluation Alliance of Nova Scotia (DEANS) and the formulary management committee. However, the division's recommendations are influenced by members of the front-line organizations, such as health professionals, hospitals, and district health authorities, and by those at the outer levels with a more national focus, such as the Canadian Agency for Drugs and Technologies in Health.

Current challenges in designing and implementing pharmaceutical programs include new and expensive drugs, aging populations, and quickly rising pharmaceutical expenditures. Delivering pharmaceutical services effectively and efficiently is a complex task that requires close attention to the changing political environment and stakeholders, along with the financial, regulatory, and educational strategies that can be used to influence programs and policies. Dalhousie's Drug Use Management and Policy Residency Program began in 2000 as one step in responding to these challenges in Nova Scotia. As the director of the program, I select residency placement sites that are receptive to the service learning model and assist students as they formulate their projects to maximize their usefulness within the placement context.

The Nova Scotia Department of Health's pharmaceutical services division is my key partner. The division determines who is eligible for publicly subsidized pharmaceuticals, which medications are funded (currently approximately 5,000 products), and the conditions for funding. As an adjunct to its administrative role, it funds DEANS to analyse drug use patterns and implement and evaluate strategies to improve drug use (Drug Evaluation Alliance of Nova Scotia, 2009; Graham, Frail, Allen, & Sketris, 2007; Sketris et al., 2006; Sketris & McLean-Veysey, 2000). I also work directly with hospitals, nursing homes, and primary care organizations.

The Drug Use Management and Policy Residency Program

Program Model, Goals, and Objectives

The residency component of the chair's program links graduate students and university researchers with decision-makers engaged in pharmaceutical policy development and program management. The residency program uses the model of community-engaged scholarship and the model of service learning mainly promoted by the Community-Campus Partnerships for Health. Boyer and his collaborators (Boyer, 1996, 1990; ASPH Council of Public Health Practice Coordinators, 2004; Ahmed, Beck, Maurana, & Newton, 2004) identify four key dimensions of engaged scholarship: (1) discovery, which includes developing new theories and knowledge; (2) integration, which includes bringing together knowledge from several disciplines to create new insights; (3) application, which includes using knowledge to solve societal problems; and (4) teaching, which includes examining both instructing and learning.

In addition to these dimensions, the residency implements principles of service learning in which the community partners benefit from a service they need. As they work with residents and their faculty advisors, they may learn new concepts that may encourage greater incorporation of research results into the policy-making process or foster new ways of thinking about problems. Residents benefit from the opportunity to apply their skills to an actual policy-relevant issue. The benefits to both residents and community partners from service learning are listed in Table 8.1 (Conrad et al., 2005). While a survey of US pharmacy schools indicates service learning has been used in some professional programs, it has not been generally applied to students who conduct pharmaceutical policy research, although such programs may have a

Table 8.1 Benefits to Residents and Community Partners

	Community Partners	Drug Policy Residents
Service Provided	1. Training of future health services researchers about decision-makers' knowledge preferences 2. Knowledge and insight into policy-making processes 3. Participating as partners in the design of research projects based on information needs for policies on drug use management 4. Real life experience that demonstrates how theory is translated into practice 5. One-on-one mentoring by a decision-maker preceptor 6. Exposure to decision-making environments 7. Assistance with communication for policy-makers (e.g., briefing notes, fact sheets with questions and answers, and verbal briefings)	1. A research or policy synthesis project about a timely drug use and management policy issue 2. Ad hoc responses to drug policy issues that arise 3. Presentations to various stakeholders within and outside the ministry

	Community Partners	Drug Policy Residents
Learning	1. Incorporating research and information into policy-making processes 2. Learning about university research 3. Learning how to apply and determine benefits from research methodologies 4. Learning how to work with researchers	1. An opportunity to refine research skills 2. Policy options analysis and policy implementation issues 3. Communicating research results to a decision-maker audience 4. Learning about trade-offs with respect to research use in different environments and for different purposes 5. Learning about factors that affect decision-making (e.g., interest groups and stakeholders) 6. New knowledge about drug use management and policy issues 7. Application of concepts, theories, and methods learned in academic courses 8. Workplace skills such as conflict resolution and teamwork 9. Ability to learn from new perspectives, other disciplines, and new settings

Source: Conrad et al., 2005. Reproduced with the permission of the *American Journal of Pharmaceutical Education.*

research component (Peters & MacKinnon, 2004; Rapp, 2003; Miller & Clarke, 2002).

Service learning joins community action – the "service" – and efforts to learn from that action and connect the result to existing knowledge – the "learning" (Stanton, Giles, & Cruz, 1999, p. 20). To provide community service learning effectively, program administrators use education theory, especially in developing skills in critical thinking (Community-Campus Partnerships for Health, 2009). As illustrated in Figure 8.2, community engagement facilitates the intersection of teaching, research, and service. With service learning, residents are exposed to two different categories of learning: (1) cognitive learning and (2) affective learning. Cognitive learning refers to the ability to apply theories and methods from research to solve real-world policy or

Figure 8.2 Community-Engaged Teaching, Research, and Service

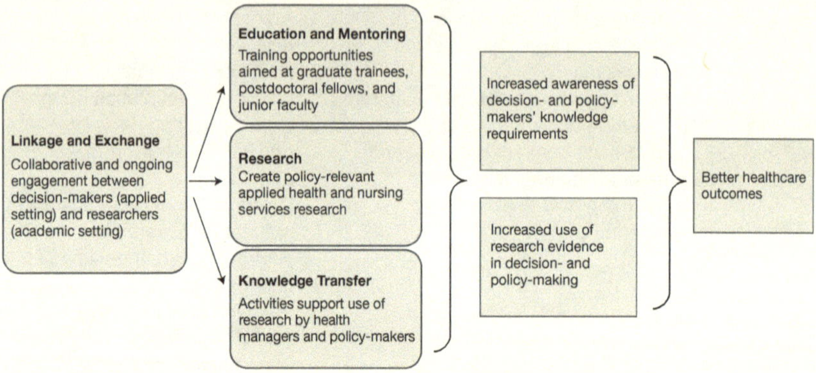

program challenges. Affective learning refers to the ability to develop new understandings and attitudes towards government, health service delivery organizations, providers and patients, and ethical and moral orientation (Peters & MacKinnon, 2004; Weber, 2006). The latter arise from examination of ethical, political, and professional dilemmas that result from new experiences (Bore et al., 2005; Jordan, 2007). Box 8.2 provides definitions of relevant terms and websites relevant to service learning.

The residency goals are: (1) create policy-relevant scientific evidence; (2) facilitate interaction among residents, academics, and decision-makers; and (3) provide residents with the opportunity to identify and use scientific evidence to inform policies fit within the service learning framework (Conrad, Murphy, & Sketris, 2005). The activities expected from each resident flow naturally from these goals, namely: (1) design and implement a research, literature synthesis, or policy analysis project; (2) communicate results orally and in writing to academic and decision-maker audiences; and (3) reflect on how decision-makers use scientific and other evidence to inform policy (Conrad et al., 2005).

Role of the Chair

I largely conduct my research in Gibbons' Mode 2 – in other words, in a context of application to include "a wider, more temporary and heterogeneous set of practitioners, collaborating on a problem defined in a

BOX 8.2 CONCEPTS AND RESOURCES FOR SERVICE LEARNING

SELECTED DEFINITIONS

Experiential education is "a philosophy and methodology in which educators purposefully engage with learners in direct experience and focused reflection to increase knowledge, develop skills and clarify values. It is a systematic approach to applied learning whereby a student is directly engaged in professional and productive learning activities" (ASPH Council of Public Health Practice Coordinators, 2004).

Experiential learning combines "learning from books, libraries and archives and learning from people with experience" (Stanton et al., 1999, p. 136).

Knowledge translation is "a dynamic and iterative process that includes synthesis, dissemination, exchange and ethically sound applications of knowledge to improve the health of Canadians, provide more effective health services and products and strengthen the health care system. This process takes place within a complex system of interactions between researchers and knowledge users which may vary in intensity, complexity and level of engagement depending on the nature of the research and the findings as well as the needs of the particular knowledge user" (Graham & Tetroe, 2009, p. 46).

Service learning is a subset of experiential learning defined as "a structured learning experience that combines community service with preparation and reflection. Students engaged in service-learning provide community service in response to community-identified concerns and learn about the context in which service is provided, the connection between their service and their academic coursework, and their roles as citizens" (ASPH Council of Public Health Practice Coordinators, 2004).

Transdisciplinary learning is "broadly constituted of a range of disciplines using an ecological approach to address complex health issues: an integrated, team-based approach to problem solving that makes a simultaneous blend and use of a broad range of disciplines to focus on a problem or issue to inform, provide guidance, and reach solutions toward using a holistic approach. The process and outcomes go beyond and transcend individual disciplines by crossing traditional professional boundaries, and

Box 8.2 (*continued*)

individuals strive to adapt their own discipline's theories and research to the needs of other disciplinary members" (ASPH Council of Public Health Practice Coordinators, 2004).

Selected Documents and Websites

- Canadian Alliance for Community Service-Learning (www.communityservicelearning.ca)
- Clover, D., & McGregor, C. (Eds). (2008). Community-university partnerships: Connecting for change. Proceedings of the Third International Community-University Exposition, University of Victoria, BC, May 2008. Retrieved 20 February 2013 from http://depts.washington.edu/ccph/pdf_files/cuexpo_proceedings.pdf
- Community-Campus Partnerships for Health. (2005). *Linking scholarship and communities: Report of the commission on community-engaged scholarship in the health professions.* Retrieved 20 February 2013 from http://depts.washington.edu/ccph/pdf_files/report%20execsumm.pdf
- Community-Campus Partnerships for Health – CCPH Consultancy Network (http://depts.washington.edu/ccph/mentor.html)
- Community-Based Research Canada (http://communityresearchcanada.ca)
- Jordan, C. (Ed.). (2007). *Community-engaged scholarship review, promotion and tenure package.* Peer Review Workgroup, Community-Engaged Scholarship for Health Collaborative, Community-Campus Partnerships for Health. Retrieved 20 February 2013 from http://depts.washington.edu/ccph/pdf_files/ces_rpt_package.pdf
- Maurana, C., Wolff, M., et al. (2000). Working with our communities: Moving from service to scholarship in the health professions. Community-Campus Partnerships for Health's 4th Annual Conference, Washington, DC. Retrieved 20 February 2013 from http://depts.washington.edu/ccph/pdf_files/tr2.pdf
- Michigan Journal of Community Service Learning (http://ginsberg.umich.edu/mjcsl)

specific and localized context" (Gibbons et al., 1994, p. 4). My research provides a platform that can help trainees achieve their goals. For the residency, I develop and manage a network of university faculty and decision-maker preceptors interested in improving pharmaceutical management. I facilitate interactions between faculty members, students, and decision-makers to identify current and emerging pharmaceutical issues. Decision-makers provide local context and current priorities, allow students to test concepts, and help implement solutions. Faculty members strengthen the decision-makers' abilities to solve relevant problems through expert knowledge of the field, methodological skills, and access to specialized resources such as information databases or computer programs. I identify relevant promising practices from other jurisdictions mainly through journals, unpublished "grey" reports, list serves, international academic colleagues, and conferences. I am able to successfully create and manage resident placements largely as a result of my cumulative experience as an engaged expert, active in both applied health services research and public sector governance. For example, I have been an advisor to various government committees concerned with setting maximum prices for patented drugs; evaluating drugs' cost effectiveness; determining the appropriateness of prescribing selected drugs to be reimbursed from the public purse; and reforming the pharmaceutical system. These experiences give me a window into the issues decision-makers face, as well as their processes and operating styles. I also work with international researchers to compare the impact of different national drug policies (Smith et al., 2008a; Smith et al., 2008b; Sketris 2007a, 2007b; Cooke, Nissen, Sketris, & Tett, 2005; Groves, Sketris, & Tett, 2003). Finally, as a result of the experiences and contacts I have made through the chair with local colleagues in other disciplines, I understand and speak the languages of different academic disciplines and can translate them for decision-makers.

One of my key roles is screening projects based on access to data sets; ethical, privacy, and confidentiality considerations; availability of specifically trained personnel to assist residents; time and resources required; and other practical considerations. I also assist all participants in understanding the academic objectives, policies and procedures, and expected outputs. In particular, I consider the development of academic rigour and the potential for the professional and scholarly dissemination of results. Preceptors have a similar role, as they explain their norms, policies, and procedures to students and faculty, including political agendas, mechanisms for transparency, and mechanisms for public engagement.

Program Function

Residents are selected on the basis of their background (university courses, research experience, and professional work experience); a written essay on their interests and goals for the residency; their career goals and references; and an interview. The potential to match their interests to those of a preceptor is also considered in order to create a mutually productive team.

Once selected, residents are matched with decision-maker preceptors and then placed in a government or health services delivery organization for a four-month paid work experience. Residents are generally immersed in the policy and healthcare environments located in the decision-maker preceptors' organizations, which allows for ongoing interaction. Preceptors serve as guides as residents learn about the decision-making processes, culture, and methods used to communicate with politicians, managers, practitioners, and the public (e.g., briefing notes, questions and answers for the legislature, and information notes for clients of pharmacare). Residents also participate in lectures and discussions on current policy or program issues.

Decision-maker preceptors are selected on the basis of having both a current drug policy or program challenge and also the authority to implement results generated from the residency projects. They must be interested in working with the residents, receptive to using scientific evidence, and willing to provide organizational support. As required, preceptors may give residents access to technical personnel, specialized internal health data or tools, administrative health data held by other organizations, or additional resources. They often allow residents to shadow them, share guidance from their own experiences, and help residents reflect on what they have learned.

Faculty advisors are chosen for their methodological expertise, pertinent knowledge, and research program direction. They understand the research process and the capacities of graduate students. They are drawn from diverse research areas because the research evaluating drug policy uses theories and methods from many sources, including clinical, social, and behavioural sciences; biostatistics; epidemiology; computer science; and economics. Some projects require transdisciplinary approaches. Faculty members need to supervise students and work with decision-makers who are involved in projects in the messiness of the real world. Where appropriate, residents may have two faculty advisors: one with content knowledge (e.g., pharmaceutical knowledge) and another with specific methodological expertise (e.g., econometric modelling).

The main goal of the project is to use the residents' skills in applying scientific inquiry to provide evidence related to the decision-maker preceptor's policy problem. The preceptor, faculty advisor, and resident develop each project collaboratively to create relevant and methodologically rigorous projects that will help guide decisions (Dash, Gowman, & Traynor, 2003). The project is often scoped four months' prior to the start of the residency. I personally meet with faculty advisors and preceptors to discuss potential projects, often suggesting three to six different topics on which knowledge is needed. Faculty members provide insights into topics from their work and discuss their research approaches. We then design the chosen project, taking into account the student's stage of training. For example, in the case of doctoral students, the residency may provide an opportunity to conduct a literature synthesis or pilot study that will inform their dissertation topic. On occasion, there is tension between the decision-makers' need for timely and cost-effective information to take action and academics' need for methodologically rigorous projects that are generalizable and publishable (Lomas, 2000a, 2000b; Roos & Shapiro, 1999; Huberman, 1990; Lavis et al., 2003a, 2003b). In these situations, the various expectations of residents, preceptors, and faculty advisors need to be managed with goals that are realistic and achievable. Of course, in most cases the residency project is just one component of a decision-makers' policy or program evaluation, and so it requires coordination with other approaches.

Projects may focus on any of three types of knowledge creation: individual study; knowledge synthesis; or producing tools to assist prescribing and drug use changes (e.g., educational program development) (Graham et al., 2006). Individual studies have included methods such as interviews, focus groups, surveys, clinical audits, and analysis of secondary administrative data or patient registries.

The framework for the residency program is illustrated in Figure 8.3. The resident, faculty advisor, and preceptor develop a project proposal and an implementation plan aided by a program manual that describes participants' roles, learning contract templates, and evaluation forms (Conrad & Sketris, 2008). Program staff provide an authorship manual and additional reading. If required, an ethics

Figure 8.3 Residency Framework

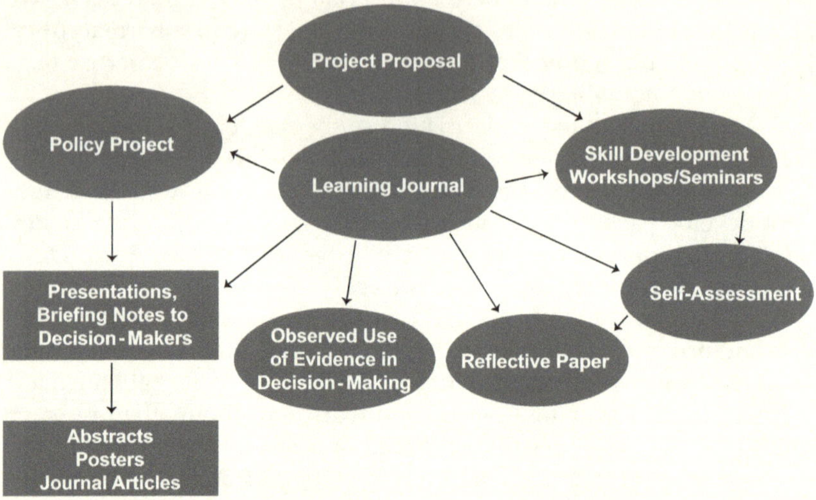

Adapted with permission from Conrad, Murphy, & Sketris, 2005.

committee application often begins before the residency project can be implemented. Residents and other team members, if interested, also participate in university-based sessions (e.g., employing reflective journals and portfolios, conducting literature database searches and synthesis, preparing ethics applications, policy analysis, writing briefing notes, or media training). Many residents might not have had access to these skills through their academic programs. Reflective learning, a key component of the residency program, is achieved through a two-pronged approach: (1) during the program, residents document experiences and thoughts as journal entries, and work to make sense of the information presented and challenges in the field in discussions with their cohort of residents and others; (2) at the end of the program, each resident prepares a reflective paper on their residency activities for their portfolio (Plaza, Draugalis, Slack, Skrepnek, & Sauer, 2007). I monitor project progress and make adjustments as needed. Residents have ongoing access to the chair's resources – the program coordinator, the preceptor, a faculty advisor, and me – in person, by phone, and by email.

Each project evolves with many iterative discussions between the preceptor, faculty advisor, and resident to define the scope and implementation plan, discuss preliminary findings, and determine how to disseminate the final results. During the early stages of the project, residents are encouraged to produce and present a briefing note that usually contains background on the need for the project and the approach chosen to provide awareness within the broader host organization. Residents may produce and present a second briefing note to the host organization with preliminary or final results. This is followed by a paper of up to twenty-five pages, or a draft manuscript with both a one- and three-page summary that follow CHSRF's communication model, which the resident gives to the host organization, and an oral presentation to the broader community at the end of the program (Canadian Health Services Research Foundation, 2009). Some residents also prepare questions and answers for the health minister or contribute to government media releases. Verbal presentations have included medical rounds, individual briefings of government officials, and presentations to senior provincial government committees, provincial departmental committees, and provincial programs.

For a number of residents, what starts as an in-house grey document and briefing notes can, over time, become an abstract published at an academic meeting, a peer-reviewed journal article, a summary and critique in a database of evidence synthesis, or an entry in a compilation of Canadian prescribing projects or pharmacy practice research database. However, we need further innovation in our dissemination approaches if we are to close the research-to-practice gap (Graham & Tetroe, 2007).

Residency Program Progress to Date

Thirty students have completed the residency program over the seven-year period; 47 per cent had prior healthcare experience (eight pharmacists, four physicians, one occupational therapist, and one nurse). They were engaged in the following graduate training programs at Dalhousie and Saint Mary's University: master in community health and epidemiology (13); master in health informatics (5); master in economics (2); master in health services administration and law (1); master in applied health services research (1); doctorate programs (7); and fellowships (1). Seventeen residents were placed at the Nova Scotia Department of Health and thirteen at health service delivery organizations. Faculty advisors have been drawn from Dalhousie University Faculty of Health Professions (College of Pharmacy, School of Nursing),

Faculty of Management (School of Business Administration), Faculty of Science (Department of Economics), Faculty of Computer Science, Faculty of Medicine (Community Health and Epidemiology, Division of Continuing Medical Education, Department of Family Medicine), Department of Medicine (Gastroenterology, Endocrinology), and Saint Mary's University (Department of Psychology).

Residents build skills and insights from project work. They may gain insight into their fit with a possible career focus (e.g., within a university, private sector, service delivery organization, or public policy environment). The experience may also pay dividends later in the residents' careers (e.g., through program-established relationships with local, national, and international researchers and public sector officials). These dividends extend to the university as residents take their places in research, academic, public, or private institutions.

The faculty members involved in the residency program have opportunities to meet with and develop research partnerships in the community. They might access new data sources and develop new research programs. Some research funding organizations require community partnerships; thus, the residency program may allow faculty to build partnerships and pilot data required for such funding sources.

Decision-makers gain access to graduate trainees to help them solve a real-world problem. The results may help inform a policy decision or provide a new way of looking at a problem. Sometimes the methods the residency project employs can be put to other uses.

The residents, preceptors, and faculty involved in the residency program identify its immediate benefits at the end of each cohort; however, the more significant benefits can be identified only with a longitudinal approach that follows the key players, and even then the spill-over benefits to communities of practice are difficult to identify.

Case Studies

The chair's program is a story of relationships fostered, research initiatives developed, and, in some cases, drug policies impacted. During the program, I worked with residents and chair partners to examine various pharmaceutical policies issues. While a multitude of challenges exist, we focused on doable projects that fit within the context of the decision-maker preceptors, and often made incremental changes. In this section, I discuss two cases, each based on one or more residency projects, as illustrations of the challenges of implementing service learning in policy environments where interests are numerous and important, such as in drug policy. The first case illustrates the difficulty in overcoming professional norms and prescribing habits, even when gold-standard evidence is available. The second case illustrates the difficulty in implementing a health technology when research results are not convergent and evidence is still incomplete.

Case Study One: Delivering Respiratory Drugs – Overcoming Professional Norms and Habits

This case study on the delivery of respiratory drugs for lung disease has several components: proving a superior treatment, speeding its adoption into practice, and evaluating the effect of that adoption. This is a common situation that arises as newer, superior treatments displace established practices. This case focuses on the comparison of two methods of delivery of respiratory drugs for asthma and chronic obstructive lung diseases, namely inhaled respiratory drugs delivered by nebulization (masks) and metered dose inhalers (puffers).

I worked with other researchers and trainees to evaluate specific components of the interventions that promote portable inhaler use. The components evaluated included health services, physicians' prescribing, pharmacists' dispensing, and patients' using of medications. The evaluations and dissemination of the results occurred over eight years as we assembled and updated literature, evaluated various components of the interventions, and determined their long-term impact. Various methods of evaluation were needed. I worked with decision-makers to involve trainees in computer science, epidemiology, emergency medicine, and pharmacy. Faculty working on these projects came from disciplines such as medicine, pharmacy, epidemiology, biostatistics, adult education, and computer science. The policies and programs related to inhaled respiratory medications were developed by several decision-makers: the Nova Scotia Department of Health's Pharmaceutical Services, the division of emergency medicine at the Izaak Walton Killam Health Centre (a paediatric university teaching hospital), and the pharmacy department at the Queen Elizabeth II Health Sciences Centre (a general university teaching hospital).

The scientific evidence. Inhaled therapy for respiratory disease can be delivered by nebulization, a portable metered dose inhaler (MDI), or a portable dry power inhaler (DPI) (Williams, 2006; Dolovich et al., 2005). Spacer devices, or holding chambers, deposit drug particles deep into patients' lungs, where they are most effective. They also help patients time their breathing correctly, and help prevent drug particles from remaining in the mouth and throat.

The spacer device was first marketed in 1983. In the 1980s, small studies showed the equivalency of nebulizers and portable inhalers (Jasper, Mohsenifar, Kahan, Goldberg, & Koerner, 1987; Turner, Patel, Ginsburg, & FitzGerald, 1997). In the 1990s, consensus panels and clinical practice guidelines began to recommend portable inhalers (Boulet et al., 1999; O'Donnell et al., 2003; Dolovich et al., 2005). The Cochrane database of systematic reviews (Cates, Bestall, & Adams, 2001; Cates, Crilly, & Rowe, 2006) has recommended the preferential use of portable inhalers since 1997. For example, in children over two years of age, the MDI used with a spacer device did not change hospital admission rates or lung function tests when compared to nebulization and reduced emergency department visits by twenty-eight minutes (Cates et al., 2006). The evidence, while consistent, was not complete for some age groups or disease conditions. For example, the 2006 Cochrane review dealt only with asthma. In addition, treatment guidelines were not updated yearly and relied on expert opinion in many areas where clinical trial evidence was limited. They rarely included information on reasons for physician prescribing, patient preferences, or cost-effectiveness (Graham et al., 2001). Additionally, some guidelines were from the United States, which has a different healthcare system.

As end users begin to apply growing scientific evidence, they might be able to determine which drug to prescribe in what quantity for a specific patient or patient group, as well as improve efficacy and increase cost-effectiveness. Nevertheless, biological uncertainty exists and means that, for many prescribing decisions, medicine remains both an art and a science.

MDIs used with spacer devices are now believed to be as effective as nebulization, as they cause less bacterial contamination and are more convenient to use. A patient's inhalation technique, while still a factor, is less important. MDIs used with spacer devices deposit less drug in the mouth and throat than portable inhalers alone. However, adding spacer devices increases costs and decreases convenience (Williams, 2006). In hospitals, there is also concern about the safety and feasibility of reusing spacer devices (Williams, 2006). DPIs are breath activated but require moderate to high inspiration. Nebulizers benefit patients who are less able to coordinate other devices and who require high doses (Williams, 2006). In other words, there are tradeoffs to each solution.

The cost of respiratory medications and their delivery devices depends on the type and dose of drug; the type, size, and geographic location of the provider (which could be community pharmacy, home care, nursing home, or hospital); and the government purchasing contracts. The cost of administration of the medication in a hospital includes administrative and personnel costs (e.g., nurses, pharmacists, respiratory technologists) for prescribing, dispensing, administering, and educating patients. At the Queen Elizabeth Health Sciences Centre in Halifax, a one-week supply of wet nebulization (including the drug and supplies) cost $167, versus $28 for a portable inhaler plus a holding chamber (Lowe, Lummis, Zhang, & Sketris, 2008).

Response to this evidence. Despite the evidence of ease of use and cost-effectiveness, there is still limited uptake of portable inhalers. In a Canadian survey, 86 per cent of paediatric emergency physicians felt the evidence was strong enough to justify switching clinical practice to use a portable inhaler plus a spacer device as first line therapy, yet 80 per cent of academic paediatric emergency departments surveyed continued to use nebulization routinely (Osmond et al., 2006).

In 2000, DEANS launched an initiative to decrease the use of nebulization. At that time, approximately 5,000 Nova Scotia senior pharmacare beneficiaries used this delivery method (Sketris & McLean-Veysey, 2000). Changing practice to favour inhalers involved a multi-pronged campaign that included information and financial reward structures. The pharmaceutical services division of the Department of Health met with fifteen respiratory drug and device manufacturers to let them know of the drive to move from nebulized respiratory therapy to portable inhalers. DEANS coordinated education and produced newsletters, brochures, and educational programs to teach health professionals and patients about the benefits and use of portable inhalers. The Department of Health also used financial incentives (pharmacists' professional fee to encourage the uptake of spacer devices and the proper use of portable inhalers), formulary administrative restrictions (limiting the use of nebulizers to specified patients), and patient payment mechanisms (making the spacer device an insured benefit). The pharmaceutical services division's reimbursement criteria were designed to limit therapy to certain conditions and inform clinicians about the appropriate and cost-effective prescribing of these drugs. The division also negotiated the pharmacists' professional fee for counselling patients on the proper use of the spacer device with the Pharmacy Association of Nova Scotia.

As a member of DEANS, I worked with colleagues and the chair's trainees on the development and implementation of some of the interventions' evaluations, with which residents were involved. DEANS planned and partly funded the evaluations, which looked at the effect of the switch from nebulizers to portable inhalers on patients. We used secondary administrative health services data to test for adverse outcomes. In a cohort of patients who switched from nebulizers to portable inhalers, physician visits or hospitalizations (i.e., one measure of adverse impact) did not increase (Sketris, 2004; 2006; Kephart, Sketris, Bowles, Richard, & Cooke, 2005; 2008). We also evaluated individual physicians' requests for patients to continue to receive publicly subsidized nebulized therapy, and found that 30 per cent of patient's clinical conditions fell outside of the pharmacare-stated reimbursement guidelines. The guidelines were subsequently changed to allow for situations where patients may have difficulty using inhalers, such as in palliative care (Bowles, Sketris, Kephart, & Drug Evaluation Alliance of Nova Scotia, 2007).

We evaluated the impact of a hospital-wide educational initiative at the Queen Elizabeth Health Sciences Centre to decrease the use of nebulizers (Sketris, Kephart, Bowles, Murphy et al., 2005; Sketris, Frail, McLean-Veysey, Kephart et al., 2006). We conducted a time-series analysis of the use of inhalers and spacer devices from two years before to five years after the intervention was conducted. We found that the intervention had limited effect. Respiratory medication and spacer use increased significantly but the use of nebulizers did not change (Lowe et al., 2008).

We examined pharmacists' response to a new fee and fee claims process for those who dispensed the spacer device and provided patient advice (Murphy, MacKinnon, Flanagan, Bowles, & Sketris, 2005, 2008). Using a survey, we examined factors that predisposed, enabled, and reinforced pharmacists' billing of the professional fees for the initiative. We found that a cumbersome, time-consuming billing process was the largest barrier to providing and documenting education related to the spacer device, and we subsequently changed this process (Murphy et al., 2005).

One resident's experience. These earlier studies allowed an excellent set-up for a residency experience. The resident, who was doing a master's in health informatics, was also an emergency room physician at the local paediatric hospital. The emergency department knew of the evidence about wet nebulization and also about a smart practice in another location. Using individual interviews and focus groups, the resident and her team examined health professionals' perceptions of respiratory drug delivery methods and factors associated with the use or non-use of portable inhalers with spacer devices in two Canadian emergency departments. She discovered that resistance to portable inhalers stemmed from perceived increased workload, increased institutional equipment costs, misinformation about the superiority of nebulization, and inter-professional conflict related to reallocation of responsibilities; for example, nurses were concerned they would lose their chest auscultation skills if respiratory therapists were routinely involved in care for these patients (Hurley, Sargeant, Duffy, Sketris, Sinclair, & Ducharme, 2008; Hurley et al., 2007a; Hurley et al., 2007b).

In an editorial following the publication of this study, Robert Wears compared the concept of knowledge translation from academics to experienced practitioners in the field to the "rhetoric of colonialism ... in which the imperial masters saw a need to bring a simplified version of western civilisation to childlike locals" (Wears, 2008). In our response to the editorial, we noted that we were working with emergency room physicians who were attempting to understand barriers to using portable inhalers in their own practice (Sargeant et al., 2008). The paediatric emergency department has since used these results to change their policy.

The switch from delivery of respiratory medication by nebulization to portable inhalers with spacers was not harmful at the population level. At the individual patient level, there was variability between identifiable subgroups who had difficulty using inhalers. A decade later, while much progress has been made, there remains the potential to provide respiratory medications more cost effectively to many patients in Nova Scotia.

An ongoing series of projects and dissemination strategies have helped continue the uptake of portable inhalers for respiratory medications. Researchers demonstrated their ability to successfully complete evaluations in the midst of professional resistance to change and operational challenges, and to negotiate different opinions on how evaluations were to take place, among other accomplishments.

Case Study Two: Variation in Uptake of Monitoring Response to Drug Therapy in Absence of Gold-Standard Evidence

In 2008, close to 2.5 million Canadians had diabetes, and 90 per cent of cases were type 2 (Public Health Agency of Canada, 2011). Several residents examined the patterns of self-monitoring of blood glucose, or "the measurement of the concentration of glucose in the blood by people with diabetes in their daily environments," using glucose metres and test strips (Institute of Health Economics, 2006). Patients monitor glucose levels not only to document glucose control, but also so physicians may adjust their prescriptions and other therapeutic components such as lifestyle, diet, and physical activity. In Nova Scotia, the government spent over $6 million on glucose test strips in the 2005 fiscal year, making them one of the top expenditures in the Nova Scotia drug program (Sanyal et al., 2008a; Sanyal et al., 2008b; Sanyal et al., 2007a; Sanyal et al., 2007b).

A recent Canadian consensus conference made the following observations and recommendations: "For people with Type 2 diabetes who manage their disease with oral agents and lifestyle modification, or lifestyle and diet modification alone, the research results are unclear on the benefits of self-testing." "There is conflicting evidence regarding the value of ongoing self-testing in people whose diabetes is controlled by diet and lifestyle. Evidence suggests that some people with diabetes may experience negative results of testing, including discouragement and feelings of depression." "The impact of insurance coverage of testing supplies is uncertain." Finally, "The panel could not reach consensus on two differing approaches: removing funding of test strips in this population because of the absence of evidence of benefit, or requiring further proper studies proving the safety of removing this coverage before such action is taken" (Institute of Health Economics, 2006).

One resident was placed with the Nova Scotia Department of Health's Pharmaceutical Services Division. The division wanted to understand which seniors used test strips to monitor their blood glucose and how often they did so. The resident had been a practicing pharmacist and was skilled in critical appraisal and epidemiologic methods. The Nova Scotia pharmacare program had subsidized the test strips and wanted to determine if they were being used as intended. The project found that there were 13,564 total beneficiaries, aged sixty-five and over, of test strips in Nova Scotia. Of these, only 20 per cent received insulin or insulin plus oral antihyperglycemic agents. The evidence on blood glucose self-testing clearly shows beneficial outcomes in patients with type 1 diabetes using insulin (Peel, Douglas, & Lawton, 2007; Farmer et al., 2007). However, 80 per cent of patients who used self-testing were receiving diet counselling only or diet counselling and oral medications. In both situations evidence for benefit is unclear. These 13,000 senior beneficiaries with type 2 diabetes used up to twelve strips per day (rather than the generally recommended four) with a mean annual cost of $615 per beneficiary. This project was published in an open access journal and had over 800 downloads (Sanyal et al., 2008b).

As a follow-up to this project, we decided to examine why patients with type 2 diabetes used test strips. The resident in this project was located in a healthcare delivery organization, and was a psychology doctoral student with expertise in psychological theory and psychometrics. The decision-maker partners were an endocrinologist and clinical nurse specialist with expertise and knowledge in patient care. They helped develop a forty-two-item survey that used the theory of planned behaviour to study patients' reasons for self-monitoring and link blood glucose testing and health outcomes. The results of the pilot project led the resident to receive a grant to further explore these connections. Information gleaned from the survey showed that 49 per cent of participants test their blood glucose levels seven days a week and 37 per cent of participants test two times per day. When asked why they test, 94 per cent indicated that they test to know if their diabetes is under control, and 69 per cent indicated they test because their care provider requested they do so. The information will be used to design educational programs for health professionals and for patients (Gatien, Lawlor, Sketris, Ur, & Vallis, 2008).

Our Response to Challenges and Tensions Stemming from the Residency Program

In the beginning of the chair's program, I implemented new components and made adjustments as I learned to better navigate the research and decision-maker interface. A challenge for me was learning about community-engaged scholarship, which included service learning with some support from Dalhousie and the CCPH and CHSRF. I had been trained to provide individual patient care and, early in my career, had conducted basic science and clinical trials research. Another challenge for me was allocating the chair's resources between teaching, research, and service, and, where possible, balancing all three. Every year I decide how many residents to enrol in the program and how many projects we can initiate in new therapeutic areas. New topics, sites, preceptors, faculty, and students without a healthcare background take extra resources, knowledge, and trust building. Also, I address demands from previous residents and their teams as they conduct knowledge translation of their project results. I need to determine funding sources (i.e., the mix from peer-reviewed granting councils, government, private foundations, and other sources). I also need to take heed that peer-reviewed articles in high-impact journals are the most highly rated indicator of significance and quality in the university environment, but our partners may prefer other types of dissemination – which may also include rigour, critical thinking, and peer review – that may have a greater effect on policy and practice change. In addition, opportunities for knowledge translation have increased as the visibility of my chair program increased. For example, I receive ad hoc requests from government, health organizations, and other universities about mentoring, service learning, or pharmaceutical policy. I also meet with other faculty, decision-makers, and students to determine their goals as I allocate my chair's resources. In addition, with the increase in the number of residency cohorts, there is increased opportunity to examine the residency projects' long-term impact. I have attempted to capture how our research influences programs and policies in Nova Scotia and elsewhere, but have not yet done so in a comprehensive manner. I also need to evaluate how effective and efficient our educational approaches were (Community-Campus Partnerships for Health, 2009).

Providing residents with an opportunity for growth, while mitigating academic institutional and reputation risks (e.g., challenges by the pharmaceutical industry), government funding discontinuation, quality control in drug cost-effectiveness research models adopted by government, as well as decision-maker risks, is a challenge with the residency program. I give residents clearly defined roles and support from faculty, and ask them to use their judgment and to seek advice. Recognizing some of the potential challenges residents may face during their residency, I have incorporated sessions into the program where residents consider their responses to a series of situations, such as whether to accept if a drug company offers to sponsor a seminar, to provide interim results to a public disease advocacy group, or to present provincial data to a national government agency before methodological checks are completed. In service learning the main focus is a chance for the residents to learn as they provide service. The experience is not just about being a research associate.

There is also tension between staying with known and readily available research areas (e.g., data sets that are well understood) and exploring new concepts, data sets, and methods. The residency protocol requires that I determine the project scope, taking into account its value to decision-makers, the abilities and goals of residents, the availability of registries, administrative data sets and surveys, privacy, confidentiality, data security, and ethical and logistical issues.

I seek to build relational capital between preceptors, faculty advisors, residents, and me, as well as among the team members, and aim to understand and determine the potential opportunities for research. I also interact with present and past team members in other ways such as seminar series, sponsoring visiting speakers, and workshop development.

Finding the right balance between depth and breadth can be challenging. There is inherent tension in maintaining depth in a specific research area, theoretical constructs, and research tools while adding breadth by increasing interdisciplinary and transdisciplinary research. When the residency program branches out into new academic research areas, I need to learn about those areas and find corresponding academic advisors. Once they agree to become involved with the program, I help them understand the applicability of their field to the problem at hand and convey both the benefits and the academic risks of being involved in this shared enterprise. Since there are no stipends available to involved academics or preceptors, I seek to build positive relationships with them and provide opportunities for them to get credit for their work, such as through abstracts and articles in professional publications. The opportunity costs of investments in new research areas are large and the future payoffs are unknown, but maintaining disciplinary strength is key for academic researchers.

Another challenge is maintaining ongoing cutting-edge competitive research versus widely sharing ideas and conceptual models. Unfortunately, pharmacy and medical disciplines do not always encourage public access to working papers, unlike some of the social sciences, such as economics. I strive to incubate and explore methods and approaches to pharmaceutical programs and policies, and to publish and disseminate them quickly. However, the time from grey report to published paper can be long. In addition, there is tension between pursuing one's own agenda and a merged site agenda, because it is often necessary to carefully scope out each project to ensure that the right skills and resources are available for it. Academic culture fosters long-term research programs; however, neither the Nova Scotia Department of Health nor its division of pharmaceutical services has a long-term strategic research plan that could help such academic planning. In response to this challenge, I established a strategic planning process to help develop a merged site research program, with moderate success.

Decision-makers want prompt answers, but faculty members want rigorous evaluations. There can be tension between early and broad dissemination and more controlled dissemination before peer-reviewed publication. A variety of stakeholders are interested in the results of pharmaceutical policy research. Decision-makers may want to release work in progress to their national colleagues before the research team has verified the resident's work. Residents have been asked to discuss project designs with pharmaceutical manufacturers and to present to other provincial governments midway through their project. Research and policy cycles differ. In a partial response to this tension, we provide interim results to preceptors, but final publications may occur a year or more after a residency has ended.

Intellectual property rights related to methods or outputs developed may also create tension when it is time to disseminate research results. There is tension between Dalhousie University solely holding and retaining the intellectual property on one hand, and forming agreements related to shared intellectual property with decision-makers on the other. In an effort to address this tension, I seek to ensure that each project team has a clear understanding of where intellectual property rights reside, especially when a project is embedded in ongoing academic or health organization's research programs. While authorship is the most common concern to the faculty advisors, some projects may result in clinical decision support systems or other products.

Finally, there is tension surrounding the amount of knowledge translation that is feasible. Once a project is completed, I get information requests from other provinces or countries. These requests indicate interest in the project and help the team understand potential applications of methods and results. However, the chair's funding does not provide for a dedicated knowledge broker position and only limited website development support is available. I work with residents, faculty advisors, preceptors, and program staff to respond to information requests to the best of our capacity.

Conclusion

A community service-learning program for graduate students in organizations involved with pharmaceutical program delivery and policy formulation is feasible. Residents who work with faculty and preceptor guidance can learn from one other and apply theory and research methods to help solve real-world pharmaceutical problems for health organizations. However, the pharmaceutical program and policy landscape is complex and fluid. Leading and managing a network of participants takes knowledge, skill, time, and infrastructure. Project management involves negotiating topic, scope, approach, and results dissemination on an ongoing basis, while bridging differences between academic and decision-maker values, culture, organizational structures, and operating methods.

Acknowledgments

I would like to thank Ethel Langille Ingram and Michael Poulton for review of the manuscript, Jocelyn LeClerc for assistance with manuscript preparation, the DEANS management committee for assistance with evaluations in which the chair and trainees are involved, and all advisory committee members, faculty advisors, preceptors, and trainees in the program.

Finally, I would like to thank the staff at CHSRF and the CADRE program chair holders for the insights they have provided.

REFERENCES

Ahmed, S.M., Beck, B., Maurana, C.A., & Newton, G. (2004). Overcoming barriers to effective community-based participatory research in US medical schools. *Education for Health, 17*(2), 141–51. http://dx.doi.org/10.1080/13576280410001710969 Medline:15763757

Applied Management & Fraser Group Trisat Resources. (2002). Canadians' access to insurance for prescription medicines. Health Transition Fund NA202, Health Canada, March 2000.

ASPH Council of Public Health Practice Coordinators. (2004). Demonstrating excellence in practice-based teaching for public health. Retrieved 20 February 2013 from http://www.asph.org/UserFiles/ASPH_10_2004.pdf

Bacovsky, R.A. (1997). *Federal, provincial and territorial government-sponsored drug plans and drug databases. Background information prepared for the conference on National Approaches to Pharmacare.* Alberta: Integra Consulting.

Bore, M., Munro, D., Kerridge, I., & Powis, D. (2005, Mar). Selection of medical students according to their moral orientation. *Medical Education, 39*(3), 266–75. http://dx.doi.org/10.1111/j.1365-2929.2005.02088.x Medline:15733162

Boulet, L.P., Becker, A., Bérubé, D., Beveridge, R., Ernst, P., & Canadian Asthma Consensus Group. (1999). Canadian asthma consensus report, 1999. *Canadian Medical Association Journal, 161*(11 Suppl), S1–S61. Medline:10906907

Bowles, S.K., Sketris, I., Kephart, G., & Drug Evaluation Alliance of Nova Scotia. (2007). Use of wet nebulized inhaled respiratory medications under criteria-based reimbursement guidelines in a publicly funded seniors' pharmacare program in Nova Scotia, Canada. *The American Journal of Geriatric Pharmacotherapy, 5*(2), 120–8. http://dx.doi.org/10.1016/j.amjopharm.2007.05.003 Medline:17719514

Boyer, E.L. (1990). *Scholarship reconsidered.* Princeton, NJ: Princeton University Press.

Boyer, E.L. (1996). The scholarship of engagement. *Journal of Public Service and Outreach, 1*(1), 11–20. Retrieved 20 February 2013 from http://0-sas.wcu.edu.wncln.wncln.org/webfiles/pdfs/the_scholarship_of_engagement_-_boyer.pdf

Canadian Health Services Research Foundation. (2009). Communication notes: Reader friendly writing 1:3:25. Retrieved 20 February 2013 from http://www.cfhi-fcass.ca/publicationsandresources/resourcesandtools/communicationnotes/10-06-01/d497a465-5398-4ec8-addf-d7cbf86b1e43.aspx

Canadian Institute for Health Information. (2006). Drug expenditure in Canada: 1985 to 2005. Retrieved 20 February 2013 from http://publications.gc.ca/pub?id=295285&sl=0

Canadian Institute for Health Information. (2009). Drug expenditure in Canada: 1985 to 2008. Retrieved 20 February 2013 from http://publications.gc.ca/collections/collection_2009/icis-cihi/H115-27-2008E.pdf

Cates, C.J., Bestall, J., & Adams, N. (2001). Holding chambers versus nebulisers for inhaled steroids in chronic asthma. *Cochrane Database of Systematic Reviews* (Issue 1), CD001491, 1–21. http://dx.doi.org/10.1002/14651858.CD001491

Cates, C.J., Crilly, J.A., & Rowe, B.H. (2006). Holding chambers (spacers) versus nebulizers for beta-agonist treatment of acute asthma. *Cochrane Database of Systematic Reviews 2006* (Issue 2), 1–101. http://dx.doi.org/10.1002/14651858.CD000052.pub2

Community-Campus Partnerships for Health. (2004). A service-learning partnership that focuses on shaping policy and decision-making skills. Retrieved 20 February 2013 from http://depts.washington.edu/ccph/featuredmember-0803.html

Community-Campus Partnerships for Health. (2005). *Linking scholarship and communities: Report of the commission on community-engaged scholarship in the health professions.* Retrieved 20 February 2013 from http://depts.washington.edu/ccph/pdf_files/Report%20ExecSumm.pdf

Community-Campus Partnerships for Health. (2009). Community engaged scholarship. Retrieved 20 February 2013 from http://depts.washington.edu/ccph/scholarship.html

Community-Campus Partnerships for Health. CCPH consultancy network. Retrieved from http://depts.washington.edu/ccp/mentor.html

Conrad, P., Murphy, J., Sketris, I.S. (2005). Instructional design and assessment. Drug use management and policy residency: A service-learning application. *American Journal of Pharmaceutical Education, 69*(5), 1–10.

Conrad, P., & Sketris, I. (2008). *Drug use management and policy residency program manual.* Halifax, NS: College of Pharmacy, Dalhousie University.

Cooke, C.A., Nissen, L., Sketris, I.S., & Tett, S.E. (2005). Quantifying the use of the statin antilipemic drugs: Comparisons and contrasts between Nova Scotia, Canada, and Queensland, Australia. *Clinical Therapeutics, 27*(4), 497–508. http://dx.doi.org/10.1016/j.clinthera.2005.04.009 Medline:15922822

Dash, P., Gowman, N., & Traynor, M. (2003). Increasing the impact of health services research. *British Medical Journal, 327*(7427), 1339–41. http://dx.doi.org/10.1136/bmj.327.7427.1339 Medline:14656847

Dolovich, M.B., Ahrens, R.C., Hess, D.R., Anderson, P., Dhand, R., Rau, J.L., ... , & American College of Asthma, Allergy, and Immunology. (2005). Device selection and outcomes of aerosol therapy: Evidence-based guidelines. American College of Chest Physicians/American College of Asthma, Allergy, and Immunology. *Chest, 127*(1), 335–71. http://dx.doi.org/10.1378/chest.127.1.335 Medline:15654001

Drug Evaluation Alliance of Nova Scotia. (2009). Drug Evaluation Alliance of Nova Scotia. Retrieved from http://www.gov.ns.ca/health/Pharmacare/committees/deans.asp

Farmer, A., Wade, A., Goyder, E., Yudkin, P., French, D., Craven, A., ... , & Neil, A. (2007). Impact of self monitoring of blood glucose in the management of patients with non-insulin treated diabetes: Open parallel group randomised trial. *BMJ (Clinical Research Ed.), 335*(7611), 132–40. http://dx.doi.org/10.1136/bmj.39247.447431.BE Medline:17591623

Freund, D.A., Willison, D., Reeher, G., Cosby, J., Ferraro, A., & O'Brien, B. (2000). Outpatient pharmaceuticals and the elderly: Policies in seven nations. *Health Affairs, 19*(3), 259–66. http://dx.doi.org/10.1377/hlthaff.19.3.259 Medline:10718022

Gatien, B., Lawlor, D., Sketris, I., Ur, E., & Vallis, M. (2008). *Self monitoring of blood glucose in type 2 diabetes: A Nova Scotia patient survey.* Presented at the Canadian Diabetes Association, Montreal, QC.

Gibbons, M., Limoges, C., Nowotny, H., Schwartzman, S., Scott, P., & Trow, M. (1994). *The new production of knowledge: The dynamics of science and research in contemporary societies.* London, UK: Sage Publications.

Graham, I.D., Beardall, S., Carter, A.O., Glennie, J., Hébert, P.C., Tetroe, J.M., ... , & Anderson, G.M. (2001). What is the quality of drug therapy clinical practice guidelines in Canada? *Canadian Medical Association Journal, 165*(2), 157–63. Medline:11501454

Graham, I.D., Logan, J., Harrison, M.B., Straus, S.E., Tetroe, J., Caswell, W., & Robinson, N. (2006). Lost in knowledge translation: Time for a map? *The Journal of Continuing Education in the Health Professions, 26*(1), 13–24. http://dx.doi.org/10.1002/chp.47 Medline:16557505

Graham, I.D., Tetroe, J., & KT Theories Research Group. (2007). Some theoretical underpinnings of knowledge translation. *Academic Emergency Medicine, 14*(11), 936–41. Medline:17967955

Graham, I.D., & Tetroe, J.M. (2009). Getting evidence into policy and practice: Perspective of a health research funder. *Journal of the Canadian Academy of Child and Adolescent Psychiatry, 18*(1), 46–50. Medline:19270848

Graham, S., Frail, D.M., Allen, M., & Sketris, I.S. (2007). The Dalhousie academic detailing service: Designing an intervention on the topic of osteoarthritis. In N.J. MacKinnon (Ed.), *Safe and effective. The eight essential elements of an optimal medication-use system* (pp. 187–99). Ottawa: Canadian Pharmacists Association.

Greenhalgh, T., Robert, G., Macfarlane, F., Bate, P., & Kyriakidou, O. (2004). Diffusion of innovations in service organizations: Systematic review and recommendations. *The Milbank Quarterly, 82*(4), 581–629. http://dx.doi.org/10.1111/j.0887-378X.2004.00325.x Medline:15595944

Grégoire, J.P., MacNeil, P., Skilton, K., Moisan, J., Menon, D., Jacobs, P., ... , & Ferguson, B. (2001). Inter-provincial variation in government drug formularies. *Canadian Journal of Public Health, 92*(4), 307–12. Medline: 11962119

Groves, K.E.M., Sketris, I.S., & Tett, S.E. (2003). Prescription drug samples – does this marketing strategy counteract policies for quality use of medicines? *Journal of Clinical Pharmacy and Therapeutics, 28*(4), 259–71. http://dx.doi.org/10.1046/j.1365-2710.2003.00481.x Medline:12911677

Health Canada. (2008). First Nations, Inuit and Aboriginal health, Health Canada. Retrieved 25 February 2013 from http://www.hc-sc.gc.ca/fniah-spnia/nihb-ssna/index-eng.php

Huberman, M. (1990). Linkage between researchers and practitioners: A qualitative study. *American Educational Research Journal, 27*, 363–91.

Hurley, K.F., Sargeant, J., Duffy, J., Sketris, I.S., Sinclair, D., & Ducharme, J. (2008). Perceptual reasons for resistance to change in the emergency department use of holding chambers for children with asthma. *Annals of Emergency Medicine, 51*(1), 70–7. http://dx.doi.org/10.1016/j.annemergmed.2007.04.008 Medline:17559971

Hurley, K.F., Sargeant, J., Sinclair, D., Duffy, J., & Sketris, I.S. (2007a). *Use of holding chambers in the emergency department: Perceptions of evidence.* Presented at 4th Annual Canadian Therapeutics Congress, Halifax, NS.

Hurley, K.F., Sinclair, D., Duffy, J., Sargeant, J., Ducharme, J., & Sketris, I.S. (2007b). *Why are emergency departments holding back on holding chambers? Facilitators and barriers to change.* Presented at the Canadian Association of Emergency Medicine Physicians Conference, Victoria, BC.

Institute of Health Economics. (2006). Consensus statement on self-monitoring in diabetes: Institute of Health Economics, Alberta, Canada, November 14–16, 2006. *International Journal of Technology Assessment in Health Care,* 23(01), 146–51.

Jacobson, N., Butterill, D., & Goering, P. (2003). Development of a framework for knowledge translation: Understanding user context. *Journal of Health Services & Policy, 8*(2), 94–9. http://dx.doi.org/10.1258/135581903321466067 Medline:12820671

Jasper, A.C., Mohsenifar, Z., Kahan, S., Goldberg, H.S., & Koerner, S.K. (1987). Cost-benefit comparison of aerosol bronchodilator delivery methods in hospitalized patients. *Chest, 91*(4), 614–18. http://dx.doi.org/10.1378/chest.91.4.614 Medline:3103989

Jordan, J. (2007). Taking the first step toward a moral action: A review of moral sensitivity measurement across domains. *The Journal of Genetic Psychology, 168*(3), 323–59. http://dx.doi.org/10.3200/GNTP.168.3.323-360 Medline:18200892

Kephart, G., Sketris, I.S., Bowles, S.K., Richard, M.E., Cooke, C.A. (2008). The implementation of policy change in Nova Scotia had a substantial impact on the drug use patterns of wet nebulization therapy in patients with respiratory disease. *The Translator,* 2(1), 5.

Kephart, G.C., Sketris, I.S., Bowles, S.K., Richard, M.E., & Cooke, C.A. (2005). Impact of a criteria-based reimbursement policy on the use of respiratory drugs delivered by nebulizer and health care services utilization in Nova Scotia, Canada. *Pharmacotherapy, 25*(9), 1248–57. http://dx.doi.org/10.1592/phco.2005.25.9.1248 Medline:16164398

Kondro, W. (2007). Academic drug detailing: An evidence-based alternative. *Canadian Medical Association Journal, 176*(4), 429–31. http://dx.doi.org/10.1503/cmaj.070072 Medline:17296946

Landry, R., Amara, N., Pablos-Mendes, A., Shademani, R., & Gold, I. (2006). The knowledge-value chain: A conceptual framework for knowledge translation in health. *Bulletin of the World Health Organization, 84*(8), 597–602. http://dx.doi.org/10.2471/BLT.06.031724 Medline:16917645

Lavis, J.N., Robertson, D., Woodside, J.M., McLeod, C.B., Abelson, J., & Knowledge Transfer Study Group. (2003a). How can research organizations more effectively transfer research knowledge to decision makers? *The Milbank Quarterly*, *81*(2), 221–48, 171–2. http://dx.doi.org/10.1111/1468-0009.t01-1-00052 Medline:12841049

Lavis, J.N., Ross, S.E., McLeod, C.B., & Gildiner, A. (2003b). Measuring the impact of health research. *Journal of Health Services Research & Policy*, *8*(3), 165–70. http://dx.doi.org/10.1258/135581903322029520 Medline:12869343

Lexchin, J. (1996). Income class and pharmaceutical expenditures in Canada: 1964–1990. *Canadian Journal of Public Health*, *87*(1), 46–50.

Lindsey, R., & West, D.S. (1999). National pharmacare, reference-based pricing, and drug R&D: A critique of the National Forum on Health's recommendations for pharmaceutical policy. *Canadian Public Policy*, *25*(1), 1–27. http://dx.doi.org/10.2307/3551399

Lomas, J. (2000a). Connecting research and policy. *Isuma*, *1*, 140–4.

Lomas, J. (2000b). Using "linkage and exchange" to move research into policy at a Canadian foundation. *Health Affairs (Project Hope)*, *19*(3), 236–40. http://dx.doi.org/10.1377/hlthaff.19.3.236 Medline:10812803

Lowe, D.O., Lummis, H., Zhang, Y., & Sketris, I.S. (2008). Effect of educational and policy interventions on institutional utilization of wet nebulization respiratory drugs and portable inhalers. *The Canadian Journal of Clinical Pharmacology*, *15*(2), e334–43. Medline:18840923

Metge, M., & Sketris, I.S. (2007). Pharmaceutical policy. In N.J. MacKinnon (Ed.), *Safe and effective. The eight essential elements of an optimal medication-use system* (pp. 117–58). Ottawa: Canadian Pharmacists Association.

Miller, S., & Clarke, A. (2002). Impact of postdoctoral specialty residencies in drug information on graduates' career paths. *American Journal of Health-System Pharmacy*, *59*(10), 961–3. Medline:12040736

Murphy, A.L., MacKinnon, N.J., Flanagan, P.S., Bowles, S.K., & Sketris, I.S. (2005). Pharmacists' participation in an inhaled respiratory medication program: Reimbursement of professional fees. *Annals of Pharmacotherapy*, *39*(4), 655–61. http://dx.doi.org/10.1345/aph.1E286 Medline:15728330

Murphy, A.L., MacKinnon, N.J., Flanagan, P.S., Bowles, S.K., Sketris, I.S. (2008). Insights into factors guiding community pharmacists to participate in a billing program for services provided to patients with respiratory illness. *The Translator*, *2*(1).

O'Donnell, D.E., Aaron, S., Bourbeau, J., Hernandez, P., Marciniuk, D., Balter, M., ... , & Canadian Thoracic Society. (2003). Canadian Thoracic Society recommendations for management of chronic obstructive pulmonary disease – 2003. *Canadian Respiratory Journal, 10*(Suppl A), 11A–65A. Medline:12861361

Osmond, M.H., Gazarian, M., Henry, R.L., Clifford, T.J., Tetzlaff, J., & Percer Spacer Study Group. (2006). Barriers to metered dose inhalers/spacer (MDI + S) use in Canadian pediatrics emergency departments (PEDs) [abstract]. *Canadian Journal of Emergency Medical Care, 8*(3), 194.

Paris, V., & Docteur, E. (2007). Pharmaceutical pricing and reimbursement policies in Canada. Paris: Organization for Economic Cooperation and Development; 15 February 2007. OECD Health Working Paper JT03220024. Retrieved from http://www.oecd.org/redirect/dataoecd/21/40/37868186.pdf

Peel, E., Douglas, M., & Lawton, J. (2007). Self monitoring of blood glucose in type 2 diabetes: Longitudinal qualitative study of patients' perspectives. *BMJ (Clinical Research Ed.), 335*(7618), 493. http://dx.doi.org/10.1136/bmj.39302.444572.DE Medline:17761996

Peters, S.J., & MacKinnon, G.E., III. (2004). Introductory practice and service learning experiences in US pharmacy curricula. *American Journal of Pharmaceutical Education, 68*(1), 27. http://dx.doi.org/10.5688/aj680127

Plaza, C.M., Draugalis, J.R., Slack, M.K., Skrepnek, G.H., & Sauer, K.A. (2007). Use of reflective portfolios in health sciences education. *American Journal of Pharmaceutical Education, 71*(2), 34. http://dx.doi.org/10.5688/aj710234 Medline:17533443

Public Health Agency of Canada (2011). *Diabetes in Canada: Facts and figures from a public health perspective.* Ottawa: Public Health Agency of Canada.

Rapp, R.P. (2003). Standardized residency training. [Letter]. *American Journal of Health-System Pharmacy, 60*(21), 2258–9. Medline:14619122

Romanow, R.J. (2002). *Commission on the future of health care in Canada: Building on values: The future of health care in Canada.* Final report. Retrieved 25 February 2013 from http://publications.gc.ca/collections/Collection/CP32-85-2002E.pdf

Roos, N.P., & Shapiro, E. (1999, Jun). From research to policy: What have we learned? *Medical Care, 37*(6 Suppl), JS291–JS305. http://dx.doi.org/10.1097/00005650-199906001-00022 Medline:10409016

Sanyal, C., Graham, S., Cooke, C., Sketris, I.S., Frail, D.M., & Flowerdew, G. (2008a). *Effect of a maximum allowable cost (MAC) reimbursement policy on patient cost sharing for test strips for self monitoring of blood glucose (SMBG) in the Nova Scotia Seniors' Pharmacare Program (NSSPP).* Presented at the Canadian Agency for Drugs and Technologies in Health Invitational Symposium, Edmonton, AB.

Sanyal, C., Graham, S.D., Cooke, C., Sketris, I., Frail, D.M., & Flowerdew, G. (2007b). Variation in claims for blood glucose self-monitoring test strips across district health authorities in Nova Scotia, Canada. *Pharmacoepidemiology and Drug Safety, 16*(S2), 209.

Sanyal, C., Graham, S.D., Cooke, C., Sketris, I.S., & Frail, D.M. (2007a, May). *Utilization and cost of blood glucose monitoring test strips in the Nova Scotia seniors' pharmacare program 2005/06: A retrospective database analysis.* Presented at the 4th Annual Canadian Therapeutics Congress, Halifax, NS.

Sanyal, C., Graham, S.D., Cooke, C., Sketris, I.S., Frail, D.M., & Flowerdew, G. (2008b). The relationship between type of drug therapy and blood glucose self-monitoring test strips claimed by beneficiaries of the Seniors' Pharmacare Program in Nova Scotia, Canada. *BMC Health Services Research, 8*(1), 111. http://dx.doi.org/10.1186/1472-6963-8-111 Medline:18501012

Sargeant, J., Hurley, K.F., Duffy, J., Sketris, I., Sinclair, D., & Ducharme, J. (2008). Lost in translation or just lost? *Annals of Emergency Medicine, 52*(5), 575–6, author reply 576–7. http://dx.doi.org/10.1016/j.annemergmed.2008.05.041 Medline:18970992

Sketris, I.S. (2004, March 29). *The DEANS wet nebulization respiratory medication initiative and other drug use evaluation studies in Nova Scotia.* Presented at Conseil du médicament, Quebec Ministry of Health, Quebec, QC.

Sketris, I.S. (2006, April 25). *Evaluating a multi-faceted initiative to promote the conversion of patients receiving respiratory medications delivered by wet nebulization to inhalers.* Presented at St Joseph's Healthcare McMaster University Grand Rounds, Hamilton, ON.

Sketris, I.S. (2007a). Analyzing international prescribing patterns and medication use: An approach to assisting in the improvement of health care quality and patient outcomes. *Clinical Therapeutics, 29*(5), 936–8. http://dx.doi.org/10.1016/j.clinthera.2007.05.020 Medline:17697912

Sketris, I.S. (2007b). Guiding the system. *OutFront Magazine, 2 (2), 7.*

Sketris, I.S., Frail, D.M., McLean-Veysey, P., Kephart, G.C., Cooke, C.A., Allen, M., & Bowles, S. (2006). A multidisciplinary, multi-sectoral alliance to improve drug use in Nova Scotia. In Canadian Institutes of Health Research – Institute of Health Services and Policy Research (Ed)., *Evidence in action, acting on evidence: A casebook of health services and policy research knowledge translation stories* (pp. 107–11). Ottawa: CIHR.

Sketris, I.S., Kephart, G.C., Bowles, S., Murphy, A., MacKinnon, N.J., Flanagan, P., Cooke, C.A., Richard, M. (2005, April 5). *Evaluating a multi-faceted initiative to promote the conversion of patients receiving respiratory medications delivered by wet nebulization to inhalers*. Presented at Community Health and Epidemiology Seminar Series, Dalhousie University. Halifax, NS.

Sketris, I.S., Langille Ingram, E., & Lummis, H. (2007). *Optimal prescribing and medication use in Canada: Challenges and opportunities*. Background report prepared for Health Council of Canada Symposium, Safe and Sound – Optimizing Prescribing Behaviours. Montreal, QC, June 12–13. Retrieved 25 February 2013 from http://publications.gc.ca/collections/collection_2007/hcc-ccs/H174-6-2007E.pdf

Sketris, I.S., & McLean-Veysey, P.R. (2000). A provincial program in Nova Scotia to decrease the use of wet nebulization respiratory medications. *Journal of Managed Care Pharmacy, 6*(6), 457–61.

Smith, A.J., Sketris, I.S., Cooke, C., Gardner, D., Kisely, S., Tett, S.E. (2008a). A comparison of benzodiazepine and related drug use in Nova Scotia, Canada and Australia. *Canadian Journal of Psychiatry, 53*(8), 545–52.

Smith, A.J., Sketris, I.S., Cooke, C., Gardner, D., Kisely, S., & Tett, S.E. (2008b). A comparison of antidepressant use in Nova Scotia, Canada and Australia. *Pharmacoepidemiology and Drug Safety, 17*(7), 697–706. http://dx.doi.org/10.1002/pds.1541 Medline:18181227

Stanton, T.K., Giles, D.E., & Cruz, N.I. (1999). *Service learning. A movement's pioneers reflect on its origins, practice, and future*. San Francisco: John Wiley and Sons.

Tierney, M., Manns, B., & Members of the Canadian Expert Drug Advisory Committee. (2008). Optimizing the use of prescription drugs in Canada through the Common Drug Review. *Canadian Medical Association Journal, 178*(4), 432–5. http://dx.doi.org/10.1503/cmaj.070713 Medline:18268271

Turner, M.O., Patel, A., Ginsburg, S., & FitzGerald, J.M. (1997). Bronchodilator delivery in acute airflow obstruction. A meta-analysis. *Archives of Internal Medicine, 157*(15), 1736–44. http://dx.doi.org/10.1001/archinte.1997.00440360162018 Medline:9250235

University of Victoria. (2009). *Mission of the Office of Community Based Research*. Retrieved from http://web.uvic.ca/ocbr/about_ocbr/our_mission

Wears, R.L. (2008). Lost in translation. *Annals of Emergency Medicine, 51*(1), 78–9. http://dx.doi.org/10.1016/j.annemergmed.2007.06.015 Medline:17681638

Weber, L.J. (2006). *Profits before people? Ethical standards and the marketing of prescription drugs*. Bloomington, Indiana: Indiana University Press.

Williams, D. (2006). Acute bronchospasm from the patient's perspective: Role of patient education. *Pharmacotherapy, 26*(9 part 2), 193S–199S. http://dx.doi.org/10.1592/phco.26.9part2.193S Medline:16945066

Zed, P.J., Abu-Laban, R.B., Balen, R.M., Loewen, P.S., Hohl, C.M., Brubacher, J.R., ... , & Purssell, R.A. (2008). Incidence, severity and preventability of medication-related visits to the emergency department: A prospective study. *Canadian Medical Association Journal, 178*(12), 1563–9. http://dx.doi.org/10.1503/cmaj.071594 Medline:18519904

9 Engaged Scholarship: Building Capacity in Health Services Research through Partnerships with Decision-Makers

ALBA DICENSO

Lohr and Steinwachs (2002) define health services research as: "The multidisciplinary field of scientific investigation that studies how social factors, financing systems, organizational structures and processes, health technologies, and personal behaviors affect access to health care, the quality and cost of health care, and ultimately our health and well-being. Its research domains are individuals, families, organizations, institutions, communities, and populations" (p. 8). Health services research is intended to inform program planners, administrators, and other decision-makers at the local, regional, provincial, and federal levels about issues such as resource allocation and the governance, organization, funding, and delivery of health services. Historically, however, there have been poor links between the worlds of health services researchers and decision-makers and, as a result, the incorporation of research evidence into decision-making has been inconsistent.

Over the past ten years, there has been an important evolution in the nature of the relationship between researchers and decision-makers. We have learned that early and ongoing involvement of decision-makers in the research process is the best predictor of whether and how its results will be used (Lomas, 2000). So well accepted is the importance of this relationship that several funding agencies now often require investigators to engage decision-makers in all phases of their research (Lavis, 2006), and scholarly journals such as *Healthcare Policy/Politiques de Sante,* specifically designed to bridge the gap between research and decision-making, welcome submissions that stem from researcher and decision-maker collaborations and include both researchers and decision-makers as editors, editorial board members, and peer reviewers.

The nature of the relationship between researchers and decision-makers has evolved from a knowledge-driven model, in which information flows in a unidirectional manner from researchers to decision-makers, and a problem-solving model, in which decision-makers commission research, to an interactive model, in which researchers and decision-makers are actively engaged from research-based knowledge development to application (Landry, Amara, & Lamari, 2001). Denis and Lomas (2003) define collaborative research as "a deliberate set of interactions and processes designed specifically to bring together those who study societal problems and issues (researchers) with those who act on or within those societal problems and issues (decision makers, practitioners, citizens)" (p. 1). Quantitative and qualitative studies of researcher and decision-maker partnerships have found the experience to be largely positive, with decision-makers providing access to data sources, "original ideas," and expertise within their organization, and collaborating with researchers to identify policy-relevant research questions and better communicate the usefulness of their research (Denis, Lehoux, Hivon, & Champagne, 2003; Ross, Lavis, Rodriguez, Woodside, & Denis, 2003). Walter and colleagues (2003) reviewed the education, healthcare, criminal justice, and social care literature that examines the effectiveness of partnerships between researchers and research users, and concluded that such partnerships offer great potential for increasing research use.

Traditional research training does not typically include education about the process of engaging decision-makers in research. To begin this chapter, I describe engaged scholarship as a theoretical framework for the working relationship between researchers and decision-makers. I then outline the components of a training program specifically designed to help graduate students understand and experience engaged scholarship. In the context of each training component, I describe the benefits, challenges, and lessons learned.

Engaged Scholarship

Engaged scholarship is a "collaborative form of inquiry in which academics and practitioners leverage their different perspectives and competencies to coproduce knowledge about a complex problem or phenomenon that exists under conditions of uncertainty found in the world" (Van de Ven & Johnson, 2006, p. 803). In a recent book, Van de Ven (2007) provided a thorough discussion of engaged scholarship; much of the description that follows is based directly on his work.

Related to engaged scholarship is the concept of intellectual arbitrage, a strategy that exploits differences in the kinds of knowledge that academics and decision-makers can contribute to a mutually important problem. By leveraging their unique competencies, academics and decision-makers can address problems more effectively together than either could alone. Arbitrage is a way to triangulate problems by involving individuals whose perspectives differ, such that understanding and analysis of a common problem evolve from the confrontation of divergent opinions (Van de Ven & Johnson, 2006).

Engaged scholarship focuses on the co-production of knowledge, rather than on knowledge transfer in which academic researchers identify strategies to share the knowledge they produce with those in a position to implement it. After all, "dissemination is too late if the wrong questions have been asked" (Pettigrew, 2001, p. S61). A more collaborative form of research in which both academics and decision-makers produce relevant, high-quality knowledge is needed (Pettigrew, 2001). Engagement is a relationship that involves negotiation and collaboration between researchers and decision-makers in a learning community. An engaged scholar views organizations not as data collection sites and funding sources, but as "idea factories" where decision-makers and scholars co-produce knowledge to address important questions and issues (Van de Ven & Johnson, 2006). In the section that follows, I introduce a training program that I led from 2001 to 2011 designed to build capacity in health services research. I then describe in detail the components of the program that specifically focused on engaged scholarship.

A Training Program to Build Capacity in Advanced Practice Nursing Health Services Research

In 2001, the Canadian Health Services Research Foundation (CHSRF) and the Canadian Institutes of Health Research (CIHR) funded twelve health services chairs, five of which were awarded to nurse researchers (Edwards, DiCenso, Degner, O'Brien-Pallas, & Lander, 2002). My chair was funded to increase the number of nurse scientists in Canada who would conduct health services research related to advanced practice nursing that would meet the needs of clinicians, managers, and decision-makers in the health sector. Advanced practice nurses (APNs) are registered nurses who have acquired the expert knowledge base, complex decision-making skills, and clinical competencies for expanded practice (International Council of Nurses, 2008). They provide direct patient care and participate in research, education, consultation, and leadership activities. APNs include clinical nurse specialists (CNSs), nurse practitioners (NPs), nurse anaesthetists, and nurse midwives. There are APNs in many countries around the world. While the United States has all four types of APNs, Canada has only CNSs and NPs, with initial work underway to introduce nurse anaesthetists.

Although APNs have existed in Canada since the 1960s and NP-enabling legislation is in place in all provinces and territories (Kaasalainen et al., 2010), they are not fully integrated into the Canadian healthcare system. With the emphasis on collaborative team-based care, APNs play important roles in new models of healthcare delivery. For example, in 2005, Ontario introduced the Family Health Team (FHT), a multidisciplinary primary healthcare model. As of 2012, all 200 teams were operational, and many include at least one NP. In Sudbury, Ontario, the first of twenty-six NP-led clinics approved by the provincial government became operational in August 2007 and the additional twenty-five have since opened. In British Columbia, NPs are being integrated into fee-for-service practices overcoming a long-standing barrier to integration that this method of physician remuneration posed (DiCenso et al., 2010a). Across Canada, APNs now deliver care in high-need settings such as neonatal intensive care units, long-term care facilities, public health, emergency departments, and cancer centres.

The integration of the advanced practice nursing role into the Canadian healthcare system is a highly political topic that involves many players: provincial and territorial ministries of health, the federal government, the Canadian Nurses Association (CNA), provincial nursing associations, medical associations, regulatory bodies, advanced practice nursing associations, administrators, educators, and allied health associations (e.g., respiratory therapy, pharmacy, and social work). Medical associations who perceive the physician role to be under threat because of some overlapping scope of practice with APNs have been especially vocal (Baerlocher & Detsky, 2009; Canadian Nurses Association, 2006).

Factors such as the recent emphasis on interprofessional practice and education, public demand for increased access to care and reduced wait times for services, public acceptance of APNs, and increased demands for service related to the aging population, chronic illnesses (e.g., cancer, arthritis, diabetes, heart disease), and mental health problems make this a critical juncture in the development and implementation of policies related to advanced practice nursing in Canada (DiCenso et al., 2010b). Many contentious issues require examination and resolution, such as those that relate to regulation (e.g., prescriptive authority), certification, title protection, scope of practice, relationships with other providers, inconsistencies in educational preparation, and role ambiguity. These issues are described in detail in a ten-paper special edition of the *Canadian Journal of Nursing Leadership* on advanced practice nursing published in December 2010. Whereas there is an abundance of research in the United States related to APNs, there is remarkably little in Canada. High-quality health services research is required to address unresolved policy issues related to the development, integration, and evaluation of advanced practice nursing roles.

In accepting the chair, I shifted my focus from pursuing an independent research program related to advanced practice nursing, to educating the researchers of the future. Since it began to receive funding, my chair was co-sponsored by the provincial nursing lead in the Ontario Ministry of Health and Long-Term Care. Over time, I developed partnerships with senior nursing officers across Canada at the local, regional, provincial, and federal levels. While individuals in these roles changed positions, those who departed often continued their affiliation with the chair program in their new positions, and those who replaced them remained decision-maker partners. Engagement with decision-makers was an integral feature of my chair program.

The chair program blended several elements: the preparation of nurse researchers at the doctoral level to conduct research to inform the use of APNs across Canada; linkage and exchange with decision-makers to ensure policy relevance and the dissemination and uptake of research results; and mentoring of postdoctoral fellows, junior faculty, and affiliate faculty. Over the ten years, I accepted three doctoral students from any university in Canada into the chair program each year. In addition to completing their doctoral program requirements at their home university, they completed a number of chair program activities over the duration of their training. The chair also supported postdoctoral fellows and affiliate faculty who were leading programs of APN research. In the remainder of this chapter, I discuss the components of the chair program specifically focused on engaged scholarship. I describe the components in three subsections: (1) acquiring fundamental knowledge; (2) learning to engage with decision-maker partners; and (3) leading APN-focused research programs. I also asked the students and faculty associated with my chair to share their perspectives on their engaged scholarship learning experiences, which I include below.

Acquiring Fundamental Knowledge

All chair students were required to take a graduate course, offered via distance, entitled "Research Issues Specific to the Introduction and Evaluation of Advanced Practice Nursing Roles" through McMaster University in Hamilton, Ontario (my home university). Within this course, one unit addresses two related issues: (1) working with decision-maker partners throughout the research process; and (2) disseminating and using research findings. Specifically, the course focuses on helping students formulate strategies for working with decision-maker partners to identify policy-relevant research questions and to collaborate through to the dissemination of the findings. Students learn strategies for facilitating effective collaboration between decision-makers and researchers, and compare and contrast approaches to promoting dissemination and use of APN-related research findings. They outline plans for collaborating with their decision-maker partners and for disseminating their research findings. The unit features a decision-maker or knowledge transfer researcher as guest lecturer. Postdoctoral fellows who participated in the chair program usually enrolled in an online course offered through the Faculty of Health Sciences at the University of Ottawa, entitled "Knowledge Transfer for Health Services and Policy Research."

To practice their skills in dissemination of research findings, each chair program student was required to write a commentary for *Evidence-Based Nursing,* then a journal that published structured abstracts, accompanied by commentaries, of high-quality research relevant to nursing practice. The assignment gave students an excellent opportunity to write a concise (300-word) summary of the strengths and limitations of the research study and its implications for practice in words that were clear for nursing colleagues without a research background.

In addition, first-year chair program students (and any others who wished to attend) met in monthly seminars to address their specific learning needs. Some years, students asked to learn more about knowledge transfer and in those instances we brought in guest speakers, such as CHSRF staff involved in the creation of knowledge summaries.

Learning to Engage with Decision-Maker Partners

Doctoral students in the chair program were required to complete a policy practicum (i.e., field placement) with a decision-maker and to identify a multidisciplinary thesis committee and decision-maker partner to guide their thesis research.

Engagement of graduate students in experiential, non-university-based learning is a recent phenomenon (Sheps, Pong, Lavoie-Tremblay, & MacLellan, 2008). A number of training centres in Canada now require their health services research graduate students to complete a policy practicum. The experience is designed to teach students about how knowledge is transferred between the academic community and decision-makers, and to give students hands-on research and decision-making experience (Rathwell, Lee, & Sturtevant, 2008). For example, the Atlantic Regional Training Centre (ARTC) Applied Health Services Research Program includes a mandatory residency placement with a decision-maker organization, for which students receive academic credit. The field placement enables graduate students to work on research projects to inform health policy and/or healthcare decision-making. The projects are determined by the mutual interests of the student and the decision-maker, and are designed to meet a high-priority need in the decision-maker's organization. The primary goals of the placement are: (1) to facilitate interaction between decision-makers and graduate students; (2) to consolidate the students' learning about knowledge transfer and dissemination of research; and (3) to show students how evidence is used in decision-making. The decision-maker provides the student with regular feedback and a formal evaluation at the end of the residency. While on placement, students have the opportunity to attend decision-making meetings at their host agency (Sheps et al., 2008).

In the APN chair program, the objective of the 90- to 120-hour policy practicum was to give students the opportunity to interact with decision-makers in order to understand the policy process, identify the factors that shape the policy-making environment, and gain practical experience working with decision-makers. The student was expected to actively contribute to an aspect of the policy process by analysing, synthesizing, evaluating, and/or transferring information relevant to a particular policy option under consideration. Students learned about the factors that shape stakeholders' differing viewpoints and the policy development process from initial formulation through implementation, review, and revision.

The policy practicum was intended to develop students' skills related to the policy development process, and give them practical experience by enabling active participation in one or more of the following policy activities: (1) research review, grey literature synthesis, and policy analysis to inform policy development, implementation, evaluation, or change; (2) internal inquiries, briefings, and presentations; (3) public policy forums, stakeholder consultations, and interest group meetings; and (4) policy administration and dissemination.

The student and the policy practicum supervisor (a decision-maker in the policy setting) mutually decided the period and duration of the practicum and the number of hours per week the student could work (depending on their other education and employment commitments). In consultation with the supervisor, the student developed a learning plan and was accountable for demonstrating achievement of individual learning objectives through participation in the policy practicum. The decision-maker was responsible for evaluating the student at the end of the experience.

In my role as chair, I worked with students to identify a policy practicum supervisor; met with the supervisor and the student to clarify the objectives of the practicum; discussed the learning opportunities in the practicum; agreed on the duration and timeline of the practicum and addressed any questions and concerns; and approved the student's learning plan.

Ideally, the student completed a policy practicum with the decision-maker who was also their thesis research partner. For example, two students, who had partnered with the Executive Director of the Office of Nursing Services in the First Nations and Inuit Health Branch (FNIHB) of Health Canada in Ottawa to identify a policy relevant thesis topic, each spent a month in a policy practicum in the Nursing Services Office. Since neither lived in Ottawa, chair's funds were used to pay their travel to and from the site and FNIHB agreed to provide accommodation and office space. While there, each participated in policy activities related to the research they would soon start. They also interviewed staff and reviewed documents that gave them background knowledge related to their research projects. Among other activities, one student conducted a literature review that fed into the development of an occurrence reporting policy, and the other helped formulate a policy on the influenza vaccine. The policy settings were not required to pay the students, although some did.

The experience gave students an understanding of the policy process; background knowledge about their upcoming research project through access to documents, staff, and the decision-maker partner; and concrete experience of the world of the decision-maker with respect to the speed at which things happen (or don't happen) and the extent to which evidence is used in policy formulation. Beyer (1997) notes that time spent on site is likely to help researchers more fully understand the issues they study and the ways in which organizations frame the topic or problem under investigation.

One student identified the following benefits of her policy practicum experience:

> [My practicum] allowed for a lived experience in understanding nursing issues from another perspective (read: not frontline or community-based) and encompassing different complexities and influences that may not be visible outside of the policy environment, provided for new pathways of thinking about resolution to issues, and facilitated the opportunity to meet and work with highly experienced and competent policy/decision-makers and to network for my own dissertation research. Observing snippets of the functioning of a national department of health is a worthwhile experience for all health practitioners and provided an opportunity to visualize its close working relationship with other federal departments. I was able to see for real that the non-profits/advocacy or representative groups are listened to and incorporated into the policy making process. The policy practicum solidified my interest in policy research and analysis.

Another student stated: "The policy practicum ignited my passion about health policy, gave crucial insight into the policy world and how to best effect change, and provided me with lasting connections to policy makers."

Along with the advantages came challenges. It was difficult to create a good balance between the benefits the policy setting received from the student's literature searches and syntheses, and the benefits the student received from the setting's learning opportunities. Ensuring the balance was appropriate required clear communication – verbally, through the learning plan, and through regular checking in – between the student and the practicum supervisor.

In some cases, the supervisor's expectations were not clear or put the student in an uncomfortable position. For example, one supervisor asked a student to participate in data collection for a program evaluation that had not been sent for ethics approval; the student felt sufficiently uneasy with this that she discussed it with her thesis supervisor, who advised her to withdraw from the experience.

One student, who completed her policy practicum (in two two-week blocks separated by two weeks) in a setting across the country from where she lived, described its challenges as follows:

> Understanding and really grasping the complexity of the environment and players is difficult to do in a short compressed time frame. I just started getting comfortable in the environment and the experience was over. For students who work full time, it is challenging, both in terms of time and income, to be away from work and family. The expectations of the practicum supervisors may be too high for the length of the experience and they may underestimate the amount of time the practicum deliverables may take.

I learned a number of lessons from this experience. While students were usually pleased to visit national headquarters for a policy practicum and their travel and accommodation expenses were covered, there might have been a way to create a similar experience closer to home. This was especially relevant when students were required to be away from their homes and jobs for blocks of time. When the experience was provided close to home, students were able to negotiate an arrangement in which they spent a few hours per week in the policy setting while continuing their paid employment.

One student found herself in a situation where expectations were unrealistically high and acknowledged only at the end of this stressful experience that she should have notified me: "I should have maintained a stronger link with the APN chair throughout the process, from start to end. I felt I should have been able to carry on – seeing it/experiencing it as an individualistic activity. I really should have engaged it more as a practicum partnership and/or team practicum between three players."

Once I had met with a policy practicum supervisor and student and we had agreed on the learning plan, I usually did not check in with the student, assuming that no news was good news. Given some of the challenges that arose, I should have arranged formal check-in times with the supervisor and student to ensure that all was going as anticipated. I also should have given students more opportunity, during our monthly student seminar, to share experiences from their policy practicums to help students who had not yet had theirs better plan for them. As another student who completed his policy practicum stated:

> While I have learned to be more comfortable in conceptualizing an experience and recruiting the necessary people and resources to make that experience happen, I believe I would have benefited from hearing about other students' experiences in arranging their own policy practica. To that end, I would be happy to share my experiences with students who are just starting to arrange their own practica.

Thesis research was another important element of student training. Traditionally, nursing graduate students have identified curiosity-based thesis questions, and their thesis committees have been exclusively comprised of nursing faculty. To ensure that APN chair students understood the importance of engaged scholarship in health services research, they were required to partner with a decision-maker who jointly identified a relevant policy-informing research question and collaborated with the student on the research through to the dissemination of study findings. In addition, to emphasize the importance of multidisciplinary research, students were required to include at least one faculty member with a non-nursing background and relevant expertise on their thesis committee.

These two requirements are consistent with engaged scholarship, as Van de Ven and Johnson (2006) describe. They note that research projects should be collective achievements in learning among faculty, students, and decision-makers working together. This engagement involves negotiation and collaboration between researchers and decision-makers in a learning community; such a community jointly produces knowledge that can both advance science and inform practice. Through intellectual arbitrage, the many perspectives of researchers from different disciplines and decision-makers with different functional experiences are identified and explored. The research team meets regularly to design and conduct the study and to interpret how its findings advance their understanding of the research problem. Over time, the team members come to know and respect one another by sharing distinctive but complementary perspectives.

In order to avoid risks inherent in collaborative research ventures, such as the participating organizations viewing research findings as proprietary and therefore unavailable for public dissemination, research collaborations require clear objectives; regular communication; a focus on getting to know and trust one another; explicit attention to relationship conflict or differences in role expectations; and careful negotiation of the roles of participants, the rules of engagement, and the dissemination of study findings (Van de Ven & Johnson, 2006).

Amabile and colleagues (2001) studied cross-profession collaboration and found that creating a successful collaborative research team is difficult. They made five recommendations for bringing together a research team composed of academic and decision-maker partners: (1) carefully select academics and decision-makers with diverse and complementary skills and backgrounds, intrinsic motivation to study the problem being investigated, and a willingness to work with people of different cognitive styles and from different professional cultures; (2) clarify commitments, roles, responsibilities, and expectations at the outset and continually update them as the team evolves; (3) establish regular facilitated communication, especially if team members are not located in the same place; (4) develop ways for academics and practitioners to get to know and trust each other as people with possible cultural differences; and (5) occasionally set aside time for the team to reflect on itself and to explicitly discuss task, process, and relationship conflicts.

Goering and colleagues (2003) also stress the importance of establishing a trusting partnership and terms of engagement, and maintaining boundaries by clearly defining roles, expectations, responsibilities, and accountabilities. They note that misunderstandings due to cultural differences can occur, and that the best ways to address them are through collaborating on mutual tasks and maintaining open communication. They also point out that the "spectre of too close a relationship between the researchers and government funders can become an issue" (Goering et al., 2003, p. 17), in that researchers need to maintain sufficient independence so that they are not (nor perceived to be) agents of the government (Coburn, 1998).

A decision-maker partner in the chair's program who worked at the federal level summarized key elements for successful engaged scholarship:

> The importance of relationships in achieving success in engaged scholarship cannot be underestimated. It really is all about relationships. The decision-maker partner role has to be substantive. Not everyone understands that there is real effort required to ensure success and to achieve the desired outcomes.
>
> Moving government policy from the realm of opinion to evidence-informed policy formation requires the additive effect of scientists and policy makers collaborating to explore: (1) the right question; and, (2) the policy options that might address the question. Health care is a complex and crowded policy space with enormous potential for unanticipated negative consequences. Thus, evaluation of policy options and of government programs is of vital importance. The more knowledge we have, the better our ability to fully explore the boundaries of any particular policy problem and to propose a wider range of responses. This takes many minds, seeing the problem through different lenses, working together for a common purpose – formulating good, defensible public policy, founded on the best available evidence.

Students usually began to identify their decision-maker partner by identifying their own broad area of interest (e.g., long-term care or Aboriginal health) and, accordingly, whether the decision-maker should be at the local, regional, provincial, or federal level. We then brainstormed who that decision-maker might be and, depending on our level of familiarity with the individual, decided who should make the first approach. While these individuals were not formal members of the student's thesis committee, they were invited to serve as ex-officio members to facilitate regular communication and participation with the student and committee. The decision-maker sometimes gave small amounts of funding to conduct the research along with in-kind support, such as covering mailing costs to send out data collection instruments and establishing long-distance telephone lines to interview study participants. Often the decision-maker co-signed a cover letter inviting individuals to participate in the study in the hope of giving the study sufficient weight to encourage a high response rate.

To illustrate, in September 2004, a chair student partnered with the executive director of the Office of Nursing Services in Health Canada's FNIHB to identify current CNS roles in communicable disease management for First Nations and Inuit communities. Later, a second student partnered with the same decision-maker to examine the practice patterns and facilitators and barriers associated with CNS role implementation in the same communities. As their decision-maker partner, the executive director worked closely with the students to formulate policy-relevant research questions, provided input into the feasibility of the study design, facilitated data collection by offering access to long-distance telephone lines for interviewing study participants, and provided some funding towards the research. She gave students access to relevant background documents, invited them to meet with the CNSs in a large group forum to describe their proposed research, and delineated a knowledge transfer plan to ensure that key individuals in her office would learn the study findings. For both these students, this partnership was a good fit, as they had each worked as outpost nurses in the north in the past.

There are benefits to decision-maker involvement in the identification of the thesis topic: the student can address a policy-relevant question with a high likelihood that their findings will be used; there may be a higher response rate if the decision-maker supports the research, thereby increasing participant confidence that the results will be used; the decision-maker may provide funding to conduct the study; and the decision-maker may assist in addressing problems related to study participant recruitment and data collection, and in interpretation of study findings. In the words of one chair student:

> The research topic and research question were selected and developed to meet the needs of all those involved in the partnership. We met regularly even before the project started and throughout the development of the proposal to examine different issues (e.g., scientific value, feasibility, interests) and the relevance of the project to the organization. This relationship is ongoing and continues for the duration of my research.

Occasionally, it was difficult to find a fit between the student's area of interest and a decision-maker partner's priorities. This sometimes required approaching more than one decision-maker, sometimes outside the immediate jurisdiction, before identifying one who was a good fit. Another major challenge that students faced related to rapid position turnover, such that the decision-maker who helped formulate the research question might have no longer had the same role by the time the study was completed. This entailed establishing a relationship with their replacement, who might not have attached as high a priority to the question or who might have had different preferences for communication and engagement.

Leading APN-Focused Research Programs

Five faculty members at three Canadian universities completed their formal training with the chair program and continued to be mentored in their roles as affiliate faculty. Each of these researchers launched a research program related to APNs in areas such as long-term care, oncology, and pain management. They continued to work with their original decision-maker partners and developed new partnerships in addition. For example, two of the affiliate faculty members are co-principal investigators on a federally funded research project examining the role of the NP in long-term care across Canada, and their decision-maker partners include chief nursing officers from four provinces and representatives of long-term care, nursing home, and NP associations across the country. Decision-makers have been involved from the beginning as co-investigators in question formulation, research method design, proposal preparation, financial co-sponsorship or in-kind support provision, and facilitating ethical approval from a myriad of participating settings. Once the data collection is completed, they will be involved in interpreting the findings, developing a plan to disseminate them, and co-presenting and co-publishing the study results.

One of the affiliate faculty enumerated the following benefits of this relationship with decision-maker partners:

> Relevant questions are identified; recruitment of study participants is improved because the decision-maker involvement enhances the credibility of the study's importance; the researchers gain a better understanding of the complex dynamic political and operational environments in which these decision-makers work; the decision-makers have an awareness of grey literature that is internal to organizations and governments and not always easily accessible to researchers; they have an in-depth "colloquial" knowledge and a critically important awareness of what is unwritten in relation to policy, practice, organization, and history which add to a fuller interpretation of findings; they are extremely helpful with dissemination of study findings because they often have insider knowledge of key contacts in key organizations; they provide financial and in-kind resources; and in pan-Canadian studies, facilitate the multiple ethical approvals required.

Another affiliate faculty added:

> I guess for me it's been very exciting to be on the leading edge of new ideas and changes within the ministry and being able to frame some of their work within a research perspective that I don't think would have happened otherwise. Also, I've been able to develop linkages with others who have similar interests. I find myself now emailing new research publications off to my decision-maker partners if I think they might be of interest to them and they do the same for me re: government documents so a nice way of exchanging information to some degree.

For their part, decision-makers appreciate the opportunity to learn more about the research process. At a recent meeting of another research team, during which we reviewed the first set of data analyses, the decision-makers were keen to learn about the various statistical tests that had been conducted and their interpretation.

The challenges associated with involving decision-makers in the research process to this extent include finding ways to communicate regularly and effectively given everyone's busy schedules, being clear about roles and expectations, and maintaining the fine balance between full collaboration and intellectual independence that ensures the credibility of the research process. At times, researchers may not have as much control as they desire over how the research is disseminated or represented, and may not always get appropriate credit for the work. Lastly, authorship of articles may pose challenges if decision-makers have contributed to the work but not in ways that satisfy journal requirements for author contributions. An affiliate faculty member who recently completed postdoctoral training noted the need to set boundaries on the relationship: "One thing I found was that I needed to create some boundaries for what I became involved in. Sometimes I felt like I was a librarian doing constant literature searches during my postdoc and there was always lots of work that I could be doing for [decision-makers]. And most of it was quite interesting so I rarely said no but I could see it becoming a bit of a problem if my postdoc went on for much longer!"

These partnerships demonstrate the importance of direct communication from the beginning about roles of team members and expectations of collaboration. Misunderstandings will occur, and when they do, it is important to communicate, try to understand what happened, apologize when needed, and move on in the relationship and with the study with a clearer mutual understanding. It is important to realize that the relationship will not always be smooth. The key is listening, communicating effectively, and remaining goal-focused. As an affiliate faculty member notes:

> I think for me it would have been better to book monthly meetings with my decision-maker partners ahead of time to help facilitate regular communications. But that being said, often our telephone meetings were cancelled due to "emergency issues," so that was tough. If I could redo it I would probably hold more face-to-face meetings as they tended not to get cancelled as much.
>
> Also, my projects with the ministry tended to take on a life of their own so it probably would have been better to develop an action list with a timeline at the outset of a project to make sure the work stayed within a reasonable scope.

The researchers and staff in the chair program met regularly to assist one another with research related issues, and reviewed one another's proposals, provided feedback on data collection tools, assisted with interpretation of data analyses, or worked through the inevitable problems that arose. These meetings were also a forum for sharing ideas and experiences related to working with decision-maker partners.

In many instances, we were able to include students in these research projects. In this way, students were exposed to research methods other than those used in their own thesis research and could participate in another researcher-decision-maker partnership. We have completed a decision support synthesis about APNs that involved researchers, graduate students, and decision-makers. One student commented on her experience:

> Through the decision support synthesis, I have gained a greater understanding of the roles and concerns of decision-makers who are introducing APN roles and have developed an in-depth understanding of the forces that shape APN role development in my region, nationally and internationally. I have been exposed to different research methods such as a scoping review. I have conducted interviews of key decision-makers in my region and have coded interview transcripts. The chair program has supported students financially to attend activities such as roundtables with decision-makers. I think that my involvement with decision-makers has made me more aware of their needs for information. It has helped me to understand the range of perspectives they must consider when making decisions.

Decision-Maker Involvement in the Chair's Program

In addition to the linkages with decision-maker partners described above, there were opportunities for mutual support between partners and members of the chair program. Along with a university administrator, a decision-maker partner co-chaired the chair's advisory board. At any one time, there was a minimum of two decision-makers on the board, which had a mandate to provide a consultative forum that could effectively guide current operations and future directions of the APN chair program.

Decision-makers have open access, via the APN chair website (www.apnnursingchair.mcmaster.ca), to the APN data collection toolkit, a compendium of common instruments to measure dimensions of advanced practice nursing (e.g., job satisfaction and patient satisfaction) funded by one of our decision-maker partners. With financial support from another decision-maker partner, we developed an APN literature database, which provides decision-makers with open access to published APN-related research.

As one decision-maker partner stated: "In a world of performance measures and accountability, it is critical that policy makers have evidence to support decisions and policy direction. The APN chair program has been a key provider of this evidence."

Personal Reflections

Prior to being awarded the CHSRF/CIHR Chair in Advanced Practice Nursing in 2001, I held a career scientist award with the Ontario Ministry of Health and Long-Term Care. As a career scientist, I spent most of my time conducting research and much less time teaching. I partnered with decision-makers in Ontario to conduct research related to primary care and acute care nurse practitioners. I had a good reputation and my decision-maker partners trusted me to conduct high-quality research.

Since the primary mandate of the chair was to build capacity in health services research and to train researchers who could conduct policy-informing research related to APNs, my main focus became education rather than independent research. Consequently, I shifted my activities from 75 per cent research and 25 per cent education to the exact opposite. Given the established trust I had with decision-makers, I was able to become a bridge-builder and student advocate, and identified and brokered partnerships between students and decision-makers. As time passed, I found I was also able to create linkages among decision-makers across the country who were addressing common issues, and among faculty from different universities who shared similar research interests.

The chair program was national in scope, which means that graduate students from across the country were eligible to apply for it. Before I became a chair, my partnerships were exclusively with decision-makers in Ontario. The national mandate of the chair extended the opportunity for partnerships across the country. As my official co-sponsor at the time of my chair funding, the provincial nursing lead in Ontario facilitated these partnerships by inviting me to a meeting of the senior nursing officers across Canada where we discussed the mandate of my chair's program. I was seen as a national chair rather than as a university faculty member, and so the chair's program became a "safe place" for decision-makers from across the country to explore policy-relevant research questions related to advanced practice nursing. Decision-makers were enthusiastic about linking with students to address these questions, and I was sometimes able to develop partnerships between students from one province and decision-makers from another. This provided rich opportunities for both the graduate students and me to become familiar with APN role integration issues across Canada and, in some cases, to support the development of pan-Canadian partnerships to address common questions. This opened the door for many exciting initiatives, and at the same time created enormous responsibilities and time commitments in terms of the number of projects going on in the chair program at any one time.

The opportunity to mentor students and faculty across the country and to engage with federal, provincial, regional, and local decision-makers meant that we were able to address many more important APN-related questions than I ever could have with my own independent research program as a career scientist. The chair's program was funded for ten years, which provided sufficient time for decision-makers to recognize it as the Canadian hub for APN research. Decision-makers supported the capacity-building focus of the chair's program, not only through enthusiasm in partnering with students for research projects and/or policy practica, but also in providing funding to support students' research.

There were several keys to the success of this training program. First was a commitment to researching a policy relevant topic. Advanced practice nursing in Canada is of growing interest, with many decision-makers looking for evidence to assist them as they address challenges regarding the introduction, integration, and sustainability of this role. Second was trust on the part of the decision-makers in the chair, an individual with a track record and solid reputation as a strong researcher in the area. Third was a home university willing to share a faculty member with a national training mandate. Fourth was having graduate students who were willing to complete additional requirements over and above those of their doctoral programs in order to have engaged scholarship skills. Fifth was working with decision-makers who understood the importance of evidence-informed decision-making and who were willing to work closely with students as they developed their skills in engaged scholarship. Sixth was technology to facilitate distance education for the students and regular communication for faculty and decision-makers from across the country to collaborate on research initiatives. CHSRF and CIHR funds awarded to my chair program supported a $10,000 bursary for each graduate student, students' travel to the policy practicum setting and to two face-to-face meetings during a distance course, and regular teleconferences with chair program faculty, students, and decision-makers across the country.

Conclusion

Engaged scholarship represents an arbitrage strategy for surpassing the dual hurdles of relevance and rigour in the conduct of research. By exploiting differences in the kinds of knowledge that scholars and decision-makers from diverse backgrounds bring to a problem, engaged scholarship produces knowledge that is more penetrating and insightful than that produced by either group alone. Work that engages both researchers and decision-makers can provide an exceedingly productive and challenging environment – one that not only fosters the creation of the kind of knowledge that solves practical problems, but also makes irrelevant the argument for a gap between theory and its application (Van de Ven & Johnson, 2006). As summarized by one of the provincial decision-maker partners in the chair program: "As a decision-maker, the benefits of engaged scholarship are immeasurable. Working together to formulate the questions and to determine how best to look at the problem is a key approach to creating good policy. The partnership between the decision-makers, the students, and the researchers allows for a much better understanding by all parties, but most of all, ensures timely and realistic solutions to challenging problems."

REFERENCES

Amabile, T., Patterson, C., Mueller, J., Wojcik, T., Odomirok, P.W., Marsh, M., & Kramer, S.J. (2001). Academic-practitioner collaboration in management research: A case of cross-profession collaboration. *Academy of Management Journal, 44*(2), 418–31. http://dx.doi.org/10.2307/3069464

Baerlocher, M.O., & Detsky, A.S. (2009). Professional monopolies in medicine. *Journal of the American Medical Association, 301*(8), 858–60. http://dx.doi.org/10.1001/jama.2009.223 Medline:19244193

Beyer, J.M. (1997). Research utilization: Bridging a cultural gap between communities. *Journal of Management Inquiry, 6*(1), 17–22. http://dx.doi.org/10.1177/105649269761004

Canadian Nurses Association. (2006). *Report of 2005 dialogue on advanced nursing practice.* Ottawa: Author.

Coburn, A.F. (1998). The role of health services research in developing state health policy. *Health Affairs (Project Hope), 17*(1), 139–51. http://dx.doi.org/10.1377/hlthaff.17.1.139 Medline:9455024

Denis, J.-L., Lehoux, P., Hivon, M., & Champagne, F. (2003). Creating a new articulation between research and practice through policy? The views and experiences of researchers and practitioners. *Journal of Health Services Research & Policy, 8*(Suppl 2), 44–50. http://dx.doi.org/10.1258/135581903322405162 Medline:14596747

Denis, J.-L., & Lomas, J. (2003). Convergent evolution: The academic and policy roots of collaborative research. *Journal of Health Services Research & Policy, 8*(Suppl 2), 1–6. http://dx.doi.org/10.1258/135581903322405108 Medline:14596741

DiCenso, A., Bourgeault, I., Abelson, J., Martin-Misener, R., Kaasalainen, S., Carter, N., ... , & Kilpatrick, K. (2010a). Utilization of nurse practitioners to increase patient access to primary healthcare in Canada – thinking outside the box. *Nursing Leadership, 23 Spec No 2010* (Special Issue), 239–59. Medline:21478696

DiCenso, A., Bryant-Lukosius, D., Bourgeault, I., Martin-Misener, R., Donald, F., Abelson, J., ... , & Harbman, P. (2010b). *Clinical nurse specialists and nurse practitioners in Canada: A decision support synthesis.* Ottawa, ON: Canadian Health Services Research Foundation. Retrieved 19 July 2011 from http://www.cfhi-fcass.ca/publicationsandresources/researchreports/articleview/10-06-01/b9cb9576-6140-4954-aa57-2b81c1350936.aspx

Edwards, N., DiCenso, A., Degner, L., O'Brien-Pallas, L., & Lander, J. (2002). Burgeoning opportunities in nursing research. *Canadian Journal of Nursing Research, 34*(4), 139–48. Medline:12619485

Goering, P., Butterill, D., Jacobson, N., & Sturtevant, D. (2003). Linkage and exchange at the organizational level: A model of collaboration between research and policy. *Journal of Health Services Research & Policy, 8*(Suppl 2), 14–19. http://dx.doi.org/10.1258/135581903322405126 Medline:14596743

International Council of Nurses. (2008). *The scope of practice, standards and competencies of the advanced practice nurse.* Geneva, Switzerland: ICN.

Kaasalainen, S., Martin-Misener, R., Kilpatrick, K., Harbman, P., Bryant-Lukosius, D., Donald, F., ... , & DiCenso, A. (2010). A historical overview of the development of advanced practice nursing roles in Canada. *Nursing Leadership, 23 Spec No 2010* (Special Issue), 35–60. Medline:21478686

Landry, R., Amara, N., & Lamari, M. (2001). Utilization of social science research knowledge in Canada. *Research Policy, 30*(2), 333–49. http://dx.doi.org/10.1016/S0048-7333(00)00081-0

Lavis, J.N. (2006). Research, public policymaking, and knowledge-translation processes: Canadian efforts to build bridges. *The Journal of Continuing*

Education in the Health Professions, 26(1), 37–45. http://dx.doi.org/10.1002/chp.49 Medline:16557509

Lohr, K.N., & Steinwachs, D.M. (2002). Health services research: An evolving definition of the field. *Health Services Research, 37*(1), 7–9. Medline:11949927

Lomas, J. (2000). Connecting research and policy. *Canadian Journal of Policy Research,* Spring, 140–4.

Pettigrew, A.M. (2001). Management research after modernism. *British Journal of Management, 12*(s1 Special Issue), S61–S70. http://dx.doi.org/10.1111/1467-8551.12.s1.8

Rathwell, T., Lee, P., & Sturtevant, D. (2008). Does it matter? Decision-maker perceptions on the impact of the regional training centres. *Health Policy, 3*(Special Issue), 106–17. Medline:19377315

Ross, S., Lavis, J., Rodriguez, C., Woodside, J., & Denis, J.-L. (2003). Partnership experiences: Involving decision-makers in the research process. *Journal of Health Services Research & Policy, 8*(Suppl 2), 26–34. http://dx.doi.org/10.1258/135581903322405144 Medline:14596745

Sheps, S., Pong, R.W., Lavoie-Tremblay, M., & MacLellan, D. (2008). "Between two worlds": Healthcare decision-maker engagement with regional training centres. *Health Policy, 3*(Special Issue), 58–67. Medline:19377311

Van de Ven, A.H., & Johnson, P.E. (2006). Knowledge for theory and practice. *Academy of Management Review, 31*(4), 802–21. http://dx.doi.org/10.5465/AMR.2006.22527385

Van de Ven, A.H. (2007). *Engaged scholarship: A guide for organizational and social research.* Oxford, UK: Oxford University Press.

Walter, I., Davies, H., & Nutley, S. (2003). Increasing research impact through partnerships: Evidence from outside health care. *Journal of Health Services Research & Policy, 8*(Suppl 2), 58–61. http://dx.doi.org/10.1258/135581903322405180 Medline:14596749

PART FOUR

Organizational Transformations and the Academic Career

The chairs were about experimentation, innovation, and knowledge, and so setting up and managing a chair program was no simple task. In this section, we reflect on the seldom-discussed challenges, some of which may well be shared by all chairs and many of which were particular to this kind of program innovative experiment.

In Chapter 10, Pat Armstrong takes up the issue of managing and administrating chairs. Defining management broadly, she begins by looking at the question of time management. Universities' workdays and workplaces have fewer parameters than they do outside academe, which makes them a poor fit with standard time measurement practices and makes it possible to extend the workday and workplace well beyond a forty-hour week and the boundaries of the physical university. This malleability permits innovative practices, but it also creates the possibility for demands with few limits, especially for the kinds of researchers selected for chairs. Armstrong then looks at the management of relationships between chairs and mentees, as well as with the Canadian Health Services Research Foundation, other chairs, our partners, our universities, and our departments. These relationships can be a source of support and effective practice, but they can also be a source of pressure and tensions, especially in a context where the focus is on measurement and visible results and where participants have significant differences in culture or practice. Similarly, the interdisciplinary work that was part of the chair program can be both rewarding and frustrating. Finally, she explores some of the lessons learned from our efforts to manage interdisciplinary activities, before turning to the question of money and organizational work.

In Chapter 11, Jean-Louis Denis and collaborators Lise Lamothe and Anne McManus discuss issues related to the development of applied research in partnership with healthcare organizations and of knowledge exchange between academic institutions and decision-making settings. They derive lessons from their experiences in the chairs program that relate to the benefits of a flexible approach to the governance of such a program; the notion that knowledge use is a shared responsibility between researchers and practitioners; and the understanding that large-scale knowledge exchange commands resources, dedicated staff, and infrastructure to contextualize knowledge production and application with significant impact on innovation and organizational change. Their experiences suggest that a clear demarcation between academic work and roles and practices within health delivery organizations is necessary to ensure the pay-off of such a program. To conclude, they argue that maintaining boundaries between academic work on one hand and the practice of management and decision-making on the other allows both fields to benefit from each other.

Location matters in setting up and managing a chair. In Chapter 12, Paula Goering examines the effects of organizational context on program implementation using the example of her chair, which was located in a health services research unit within a teaching hospital, outside of the typical university environment. Her analysis is relevant to current debate and discussion about the value of embedded research units and researchers and the effect of having more distributed sites for knowledge production. She carefully describes this specific example of a chair that is a part of a health provider agency while closely affiliated with a university medical school department to explore salient characteristics of a hybrid Mode 1/Mode 2 model of knowledge production. Based on this description, she argues that the organizational factors that can facilitate or hinder integrated knowledge translation include structure, orientation, incentives, and resources. Innovations that have been influenced by these factors include the use of a consulting practice as a vehicle of knowledge transfer, the introduction of a knowledge broker, revisions of promotion policy and procedures, and the implementation of educational programs. She argues that protecting academic freedoms, balancing rigour and relevance, and gaining access to the benefits of teaching all need to be considered. She concludes with a discussion of the role of the builder: how the personal career of research leaders must fit with the environments in which they operate.

10 Managing to Manage: The Daily Practices of a Chair

PAT ARMSTRONG

Being awarded a chair brings a euphoria that is quickly tempered by the daily work of chairing. This chapter is about managing, understood in broad, rather than business or other disciplinary, terms. All of us must learn to manage our time, our relationships, our research projects, our students, and our budgets. However, the CHSRF/CIHR chairs program presented particular challenges and opportunities that together make it a qualitatively different experience. It is an experiment intended to help transform aspects of operation in universities and communities; to be a source of mainstreaming while not being mainstream, as one chair put it. Although aspects of the program are unique, many of its lessons have much broader implications, not only for those developing or taking up a chair but also for those seeking to work across disciplines and communities in ways that ensure knowledge is both useful to and used in practices.

This chapter is based on my experiences as a chair, enhanced by interchanges with the entire range of participants in this experiment. My chair is unique in several ways. It did not grow out of a particular content area such as home care; it is not located in a single program such as pharmacy; and health services were not located at my university when my program began. Nor did my chair have a pre-existing home. Moreover, in my application, I specifically rejected the notion of developing a project of my own that would become the focus of students' work. Rather, my chair is about bringing an approach that is often labelled gender-based analysis to bear in health services. It is intended to support students, postdoctoral fellows, and junior faculty who take up policy-relevant research that makes gender critical in analysis. It was built on my pre-existing connections with my partners, the Canadian Federation of Nurses' Unions and Health Canada's Women's

Bureau, but not on a relationship between them, although this necessarily changed with chair funding. The particularities of my chair influence the examples used here and may well emphasize some aspects of management that are more problematic for a sociologist at York University working in health services research than they are for other chairs. However, the intent of this chapter is to reflect on my experiences and practices in ways that draw out broader lessons for funding agencies and for those they fund, as well as for their partners and their universities.

We all bring particular histories and ways of seeing to the practices of chairing, and so to begin I set out some of the guiding threads in my work and in my analysis of managing. Defining management broadly, I then turn to the question of time management, as time has become a critical and recurring issue for all the chairs. Universities' workdays and workplaces have fewer parameters than those outside academe, which makes them a poor fit with standard time measurement practices and makes it possible to extend the workday and workplace well beyond a forty-hour week and the boundaries of the physical university. This permeability permits flexibility and innovation, but it also creates the possibility for demands with few limits, especially for the kinds of researchers selected for chairs.

After considering time, I look at the management of relationships with mentees as well as with CHSRF, other chairs, our partners, our universities, and our departments. These relationships can be a source of support and of effective practices, but they can also lead to pressure and tension, especially in a context where the focus is on measurement and visible results and where participants have significant cultural or practice differences. Similarly, interdisciplinary work can be both rewarding and frustrating.

In the following section, I explore some of the lessons learned from the chairs' efforts to manage interdisciplinary work within the context of a program that emphasizes knowledge sharing outside academe. Then, I explore the question of money and organizational work. There are particular issues that arise out of a focus on supporting students and junior faculty, as well as more general ones that arise from making decisions about who gets what according to what criteria.

Ways of Seeing

According to the 2004 American Sociological Association presidential address, public sociology "brings sociology into a conversation with publics, understood as people who are themselves involved in conversations. It entails, therefore, a double conversation" (Burawoy, 2005, p. 3). For Burawoy, public sociology is based on rigorous methods, accumulated knowledge, specified questions, and theoretical frameworks. He identifies what he calls "organic public sociology" as a form of public sociology that involves the sociologist working "in close connection with a visible, thick, active, local and often counter-public." Although much of public sociology is of this vein, he goes on to explain that it is often considered a private practice on the part of the sociologist and "apart from their professional lives" (Burawoy, 2005, p. 4).

I conceive of the CHSRF/CIHR chairs program as an effort to make academic work public in this sense of engaging in conversations based on empirical research – albeit conversations that work across disciplines and scales – with those in positions to make decisions about policies and practices. Like Burawoy (2005), the chairs program recognizes the problem of relegating this labour to the private lives of academics and seeks to make these conversations integral to the academic enterprise. Knowledge exchange, to use the term employed in the initial call for applications, requires us to initiate conversations with a public outside academe and to encourage and train students to do the same. But this task also means struggling to have such work acknowledged as part of our professional lives, a struggle that is, to some extent at least, about managing.

For me, this effort at public intellectual work has to be understood within the context of the current political economy and the location of funding agencies, partners, and universities within that economy. Like the critical management studies' notion of reflexivity, I recognize "the role of cultural conditions in the production of research" and in daily practices (Grey, 2005, p. 8). Increasingly, the business of government is business, and the criteria for management as well as for assessment are taken from business. Funding organizations such as CHSRF are expected to adopt these practices just like government departments. Universities have faced years of cutbacks, as well as years of emphasis on becoming more efficient according to business notions of efficiency (Turk, 2000). Support services within universities have been significantly reduced at the same time as new technologies have made it possible for faculty to do more clerical work. With declining financial support from governments, faculty members are under increasing pressure to seek out external funding for themselves and for their students. Located within public institutions and focused on what are still mainly public services, chairs receive public money to build capacity in ways that are immediately relevant and useful outside the university. Unlike most faculty members, we have adequate resources for much of our administrative work. All these factors influence the support and tension chairs face, as well as the strategies available to address them.

As Henry Mintzberg, McGill University's famous professor of management studies, wrote in his book *The Structuring of Organizations* (1979), universities are very particular kinds of organizations that require their own forms of management. More recently, he has railed against both the application of private sector practices to public institutions and the assumption that within public organizations one form of management fits all (CBC, 1999). Like Janice Gross Stein (2001), Mintzberg is particularly concerned about the cult of efficiency that is "the cult of calculation" (quoted in Swift, 1999, p. 18), an "obsession with measurement" (quoted in Swift, 1999, p. 18). Equally important, in terms of the public sector at least, he worries about over-specialization and the division of labour leading to worldviews that separate colleagues from one another. For him, interpersonal relationships are integral to good management. He also worries about the separation of management in the public sector from the content of what is being managed, and argues that management requires an understanding of the work and the workers, especially in the public sector. In an *Ideas* interview with the CBC, he also stresses that "the more professional the workforce becomes, the more you've got to deal with them as colleagues and not as subordinates" (CBC, 1999:14).

I framed this chapter and my chair through a similar approach. I assume that universities are special kinds of workplaces – ones where managers are called administrators precisely because they need to know about the content of the work at hand and the practices of those who work there. Like Michel Foucault (1980), I understand that governance is an integral part of daily practices. But, like Dorothy Smith (1999, p. 94), "I do not accept Foucault's view, at least its popularization, that knowledge is necessarily a relation of power." A university strives to be a place of collegial relationships not only among faculty but also between faculty and graduate students. It is also a place where challenging ideas should flourish. While management implies control, administration connotes service. Indeed, in a discussion about this issue, another chair suggested that the notion of stewardship applies. In the university context, stewardship refers to the responsibility to appropriately use and develop a full range of resources based on shared values and objectives. (For more about stewardship, see Beckhard [1969].) I use the term "management" here to encompass the full range of activities involved in our daily practices and these notions of both the specificity in the university context and of stewardship.

The CHSRF/CIHR chairs program's call for applications identified research, mentoring, and knowledge translation as the program key components, and implied an integral relationship between mentoring and research and promoting relationships between them and partners outside the university. The call recognized that the chairs were researchers who mentored and managed through research and knowledge-sharing practices – in other words, people who knew the work. In addition, the call encouraged interdisciplinary and applied work that would enhance integration not only across traditional disciplines within the university, but also across university, policy, and practice borders. It was thus an attempt to overcome interdisciplinary specialization and old divisions of labour.

Management was not mentioned in the call for applications, even though it quickly became clear that chairs have people, relationships, money, and multiple reporting channels to manage. The form of relationships between chairs and CHSRF, between chairs and partners, and between chairs and those they mentor, or among chairs, was not addressed either. Determining how to handle these managerial issues became urgent, and often contentious. It was contentious in part because the various participants began with different assumptions about management and efficiency, in part because it took a long time to bring these assumptions into open discussion, in part because chairs had different supports in place and different approaches to their work, and in part because new managerial questions emerged as we put the experiment into practice. We had growing pains individually and collectively, but relations and some lessons worth sharing are emerging with these new practices.

Time

As Heather Menzies (2005) explains, faculty face increasing time constraints due to transformations in universities as a result of funding cutbacks, new "accountability" practices, new business approaches that result in downloading work to faculty, and new technology. Faculty members now do more of their own clerical, organizational, and financial work, as well as facing increasing pressure to seek funding that will support students and to publish in refereed journals. All faculty members feel these pressures, but as chairs we feel particular strain as a result of the additional responsibilities that came with funding and with the new work of knowledge exchange and partnerships. At the same time, and particularly as these pressures became the subject of our collective discussion, chairs began to use funds and organize work and reporting in ways that became more manageable. In this section, I consider the time demands and strategies in chair work. It is important to emphasize again that I speak from a particular place, albeit one informed by my discussions with other chairs.

Perhaps the most obvious difference between chairs and other faculty is the need to spend time with, and devote time to, working with our partners. Every chair was required to have a decision-making partner from outside the university. Such partnerships are not a common part of academic life, at least not in the social sciences and humanities. Indeed, as Burawoy (2005) makes clear, such relationships have long been understood as part of our private rather than our professional lives. However, these partnerships were one of the innovative aspects of the CHSRF/CIHR chairs program. Both the development and maintenance of such partnerships take time. Partnerships require trust, and trust requires a time investment to allow people to know and understand others' limits and approaches. It takes time to share knowledge, another innovative part of our mandate. In addition, the partnerships often meant travel not only outside of the university and its area, but also outside of the country as the international aspects of our work grew. The process of both making partnerships a part of our regular working day and also promoting an understanding of this work as part of our academic contributions took time. So did helping partners understand that the chairs work with particular time frames.

Certainly, many chairs had worked with our decision-maker partners in the past. Indeed, to some extent, a pre-existing connection was necessary to qualify for the award. But the chair program formalized the relationship, making partnerships a requirement rather than an option and establishing expectations about time committed to partners. This often meant our partners felt freer to call on us to speak at events, provide advice, support research, and attend meetings. At the same time, the focus on knowledge translation with partners led to more media attention, which in turn helped create even more demands on our time. Initially, the requests often felt energizing and flattering, but after a while, they too became exhausting.

The formal recognition of partnerships and knowledge exchange also meant we could build both activities into our daily schedules and have our universities acknowledge them. We could create time by teaching less or doing less administrative work. Our regular meetings together as chairs helped us develop ways to draw limits on our time with partners, to resist the pressure to always be available, and to understand what were reasonable expectations of our time and knowledge. We started to figure out ways to explain these limits to our partners and universities. In addition, the relationships we developed with partners eventually saved time, since we had established contacts for policy work and for student research or internships. In such situations, we did not have to start from scratch; we knew who to reach, and could get our emails returned quickly. The trust we developed with partners over time made these relations both faster and easier.

The requirement that each chair have a governing structure added another layer to our responsibilities and thus to our schedules. Few regular faculty members have to address this kind of demand. Most funding requirements call for an annual report or reports at the end of the grant. But this funding also required us to have a governing structure that included people from outside the university to advise on the chair. In some ways, this requirement reflected the increasingly dominant calls for accountability defined in business terms. In others, it was intended to promote more continuous consultation with external organizations that would support us in our exchange work. Although some chairs already functioned through organizational structures with relevant policies and procedures in place, we had to develop our own policies for funding and other aspects of each particular program. Advisory boards could be part of this process, but the development took time – often more than it would in an exclusively academic setting, given the different viewpoints, experiences, and assumptions of those involved. For example, I developed policies and procedures for my internship program with input from partners who are part of my chair's advisory board. Although those policies are always evolving, they have resulted in a program that takes less time to run than it did to set up in the first place.

Added to this was the requirement to meet at least twice a year with the other chairs and at other times with CHSRF staff. Moreover, as the CHSRF and CIHR programs expanded, chairs were increasingly called on to participate in them. The regional training centres within the CADRE program provide a personal example. Working on the proposal, seeking university approval, and serving as co-director of the York program has taken a great deal of time. Such additional work frequently has us flying across the country and devoting long hours to planning and reporting.

The flip side of this time demand is the support, information access, and advice we receive. Partners' participation on advisory boards helps us plan our work in ways that we know are relevant to them. Advisory boards can also promote time limits by making demands visible and streamlining some of the decision-making work. They are themselves a form of knowledge exchange – one of those conversations with the public. The very existence of an advisory board promotes strategic planning over the long term, which most faculty rarely have the opportunity to do. As we got to know other chairs and members of CADRE better, we increasingly shared strategies for dealing with everything from administration to student funding. All this, too, began to save time. Regular faculty rarely have the opportunity to meet over such a long period with a group from many disciplines with similar concerns, and to learn each lesson together and faster than each would alone.

A similar process happened with the CHSRF staff as we began to trust and support each other. Participation in, for example, review panels and CHSRF projects meant we had access to information and resources that otherwise would have taken considerable time to explore. When I was developing a grant proposal on long-term care that required at least one partner, I was able organize that partnership with a single phone call – a much faster process than the endless calls, descriptions, and explanations many faculty members make in order to establish such arrangements.

With cutbacks and a new emphasis on making universities efficient, all faculty face growing pressure to apply for, and engage in, funded research. However, the pressure is greater and more complicated for chairs. With the focus on mentoring and working with partners came increased pressure to conduct more collaborative research. The emphasis on innovative research with integral interdisciplinary practices and exchange made the work more difficult as well as more exciting. Our CHSRF funding allowed us to support students, postdoctoral fellows, and junior faculty, but in order to attract them we needed to be producers with a current reputation in the field ourselves. This also meant applying for funding to support the research and researchers, which in turn also meant publishing. Neither is easy when the approaches are new and journals do not know how to evaluate them. The pressure is acute in the social sciences, where funding is scarcer than in other sciences and where there is little tradition of publishing with students who have worked on shared projects. There are also significantly fewer places to publish. All of this takes time.

In funding students and postdoctoral fellows, the chairs' program attracts students to these less traditional approaches to research. These students could conduct some of the research, writing, and exchange work. While in sociology this does not mean they, instead of me, do it, their work supports my writing and they take increasing responsibility for writing collaborative work that I once mainly did alone.

Success in producing publications and gaining funding, in turn, leads to further requests to participate in others' research projects. While any academic might feel this pressure, the chairs became more visible across disciplines as the program developed and as their approaches became not only more accepted but also more admired. Perhaps we felt more pressure to respond positively given our mandate and our looming five-year review. Furthermore, as the Social Sciences and Humanities Research Council (SSHRC) and CIHR moved to promote both interdisciplinary work and partnerships, other researchers saw the chairs as experienced in this kind of work, with established contacts. For similar reasons, these organizations called on chairs to serve on peer-review and other committees. Success in carrying out the mandate bred demand, but that demand in turn increased the time pressure we faced.

On the other hand, work experience and our national and international contacts made us faster and allowed us to scale up projects. Equally importantly, the students, postdoctoral fellows, and junior faculty we worked with began to be invited to serve on these reviews as well. Our mandate was about building capacity, and as we did so, there were more people around to share the work. Recently, the postdoctoral fellow with my chair reported that she was inundated with requests to review and serve on panels.

Mentoring also takes time. Though all academics mentor, our focus on graduate work resulted in a growing body of graduate students in the early years of the program, as each year more were added before the prior ones graduated. The emphasis on knowledge translation can also mean that we spend more time working with students to share research outside academe and expose them to our partners. For example, CHSRF offers to support a student or two to attend conferences each year. Selecting these students takes time, as does preparing them to attend and debriefing them when they return. Similarly, the chairs regularly bring all the CHSRF-funded Ontario Training Centre students together to consider issues such as the policy and research practicum. While this helps build strong relationships, it also takes time.

As is the case with capacity-building in general, mentoring under the chair does have rewards beyond those usually experienced with students. For example, one postdoctoral fellow's participation in the program took her through an internship at Health Canada and work with our Women and Health Care Reform Group, which is funded by my partner, the Bureau of Women's Health and Gender-Based Analysis. This work contributed to her selection by the Executive Search Program in the federal government. From her position in the Public Health Agency of Canada, she continues to participate in the reform group's activities, extending our exchange capacities and mentoring students in my program. Another woman worked in health services, but returned to finish her doctorate with me and now teaches health services at my university. This mentoring, enhanced by the financial support that made her return possible, means she is now involved with research projects connected to my chair and mentors students who are part of the program.

In sum, academics – especially those selected in the CHSRF/CIHR chairs program, who had to be high producers in order to qualify – tend to be workaholics. The awards, at least initially, intensified the time pressure on those already facing it. However, the chairs also provided means to relieve some of that pressure. They allowed us to teach fewer courses, creating more flexibility in our schedules and more time for other work. As CHSRF realized that the university structure and finances limited our access to administrative support, I was encouraged to use some of our funding to buy time through such support. This was particularly helpful to me because I came into the chair position with no infrastructure support. Also, as we contributed to building capacity through our work with students, postdoctoral fellows, and junior faculty, they have gradually begun to take over part of our workloads. As we established procedures and relationships, we were able to take shortcuts to get the work done. We have also learned to say no when the pressures became too great. We learned time management skills in part as we shared our own experiences with each other and with CHSRF. We could do such work in part because we had a ten-year time frame, which allowed for this sharing, this learning, this capacity-building, this strategic planning, and this need to change practices to fit with the cultures of universities and partners.

The lesson here is to think about time in the context of a never-ending day for academics and declining support in much of the public sector. Programs like those of the chairs come with new and different demands. There is considerable variation among universities and departments that must be recognized, but there are also some shared pressures that can be addressed. This means limiting demands, reducing expectations, and providing structural supports. It also means creating the conditions that allow chairs to share what they have learned with others, both within their own universities and also among their decision-making partners. It means recognizing that work takes time. This section is also about change over time, and the ways our priorities and practices altered in response to feedback on our experiment from chairs, from CHSRF, from partners, and from participants in the program.

New and Different Networks and Relationships

Academic work has long supported, and been supported by, a particular kind of culture and organization. As my earlier quote from Mintzberg implies, this culture is a specificity I see as valuable in creating the conditions for innovation and critique. In the context of the current political economy, however, lines between the academy, governments, and other organizations are increasingly blurred. Universities try to act more like businesses in order to become more efficient and effective, which themselves are often defined in business terms. Universities also face pressure to create products with commercial value. The CHSRF/CIHR chairs program was intended to cross boundaries – not in ways intended to promote a business model for universities or commercial products, but rather in ways that encourage outside organizations to use academic research and universities to conduct research in ways that lead to effective decision-making. The purpose is to create more formalized and integrated means of integrating teaching, research, and knowledge exchange. This is not an easy balancing act. Uniting universities and partners under the umbrella of a third party such as CHSRF can create a culture clash. Indeed, the differences between academic work and other forms of labour have created some tensions in managing the relationships that are integral to being a CHSRF chair, while simultaneously promoting and supporting some aspects of our work. In this section, I explore some of these tensions and the ways the chairs have learned to address them, while still building support. Again, I speak from my own experience, although it is informed by work with other chairs.

Tensions with CHSRF

Academics are not so much ungoverned as ungovernable. As Foucault (1997) and Rose (1996) argue, we have all internalized forms of self-discipline appropriate to these times. Being a successful academic requires even more self-discipline. Indeed, most academics are in this sense hyper-disciplined, because we have learned to discipline ourselves on a daily basis with very little managerial or administrative oversight. This hyper-discipline is required by the nature of the creative work we do, especially since we work with graduate students who are quite independent on research that must retain some independence. At the same time, this hyper-discipline tends to make us resistant to outside governance, especially the sort that requires or implies control over our time, our research, our teaching, and our partnerships. To a large extent, our work simultaneously requires this kind of discipline and resistance along with malleable offices and schedules.

The differences in cultures rather quickly became evident in our relationships with CHSRF. These relationships and tensions varied among chairs, just as our cultures vary with disciplines. However, we shared some common points of tension, which stemmed in part from the notion held by some that CHSRF's contribution to our salaries gave it the position of employer. This raised questions about what kinds of demands CHSRF could make on our time, not only in terms of attendance at meetings but also in terms of reporting matters such as time spent with students and in our workplaces.

The issue of control over our time became particularly critical when it became evident that CHSRF did not expect us to take our sabbaticals as scheduled. Here the problem was not simply ungovernable academics, but also bargained rights negotiated with our employer. Sabbaticals highlighted differences in views about who the employer was and who set the conditions of employment. The tension over this issue in particular sparked a discussion that led to some clarification of the rights we retained as professors employed by universities. We not only had the right to sabbaticals, but also to other conditions established with universities as our employers.

This still left open the question of areas of accountability and reporting, as well as appropriate demands on our time. Initially, CHSRF required elaborate and detailed reports and emphasized time measurement as a way to quantify our work for the purposes of accountability. This technique was taken directly from business and reflected the move within government to apply business sector practices without recognizing the issues raised by Mintzberg (1979). These reports, in turn, raised questions about the amount of time chairs devoted to their own research and to student work. For me, this is where the cultural clash became most evident, and such approaches raised critical questions about how mentoring and research are understood. Students come to work with me because I conduct research and I understand mentoring as an integral aspect of much of what I do on a daily basis. Students do not work on my projects in a lab for specified periods of time, but rather usually work independently at an uneven daily, weekly, and monthly pace. I proposed to support students in their work rather than primarily having them support me in mine. At the same time, students work alongside me on a variety of projects carried out with partners, and we spend many a weekend meeting or writing with them. In short, my mentoring is not a discrete, measurable activity, and reducing it to a numerical value would be meaningless, at least for me and for most sociologists. I saw such a requirement as a failure to understand that mentoring could not be easily defined in terms of any standard time frame, given the multiple ways in which I interact with students and especially in the exchange work of the chair. From my perspective, this form represented a failure to understand that our work is not nine-to-five or easily segmented into accountable pieces of the sort used in business. I perceived it as an unwarranted intrusion into university affairs by those basing their request on business principles.

While not all chairs necessarily shared my concerns about time reporting, we all experienced the weight of reporting in cumbersome detail as we recognized the pressure on CHSRF to keep us visibly accountable. The weight and nature of the reporting became a problem, at least for some chairs. In addition, when CHSRF asked for details on our students' activities before and after graduation, we questioned the ethics of supplying such information without students' consent – another indication of cultural clash. Our resistance was not to accountability per se, but rather to the forms it took and the failure to understand university practices. However, we were able to work out a simpler way of reporting and an ethical way of recording student participation once we understood the issues and the differing perspectives on them.

The content of meetings was another area of tension that emphasized differences between chairs and CHSRF. Initially, much of our time was spent either on bureaucratic issues such as reporting rules provided by staff, or with outside experts on matters such as mentoring. Chairs wanted more time to learn from each other, and more time to discuss the content of their work. Gradually, the meetings shifted in response, and we have discovered that we have much to learn from each other as well as from CHSRF. We have learned about techniques for managing management issues, a critical step in managing to manage. We have also learned that, collectively, we have the expertise we require to carry out the work. We just need to share what we know.

It took a while to come to this shared understanding, especially since initially we met only in the presence of CHSRF staff and we were reluctant or even unable to raise matters of governance. At the same time, CHSRF required, and provided resources for, regular meetings and so made it possible for us to begin to work together and to realize we needed time together. Once we were able to meet alone, it was possible for the chairs to develop a better understanding of our individual and collective concerns. Such discussions, in turn, allowed us to articulate our concerns to CHSRF and allowed CHSRF to respond appropriately. The need to share and articulate concerns through separate meetings of funder and recipients took a while to learn but was worth learning.

It also took time to learn the lessons about the problems created by applying accounting mechanisms taken from other sectors to universities. The tensions with CHSRF highlighted differences both within university departments and between universities and external organizations operating under rules and assumptions increasingly used in business.

Tensions with Partners

We did not feel tensions based on cultural differences in workplace, schedules, and governance only in our encounters with CHSRF; we also felt them in our relationships with partners. While governance issues were not the same as they were with CHSRF, there were still tensions around who could ask whom to do what and when. One of my partners, for example, initially expected me to be available on call to review papers submitted to them and expected to vet my presentations in advance. There are also questions about which research should be done and the uses to which it should be put. Decision-makers do not necessarily want to ask or answer the same questions as an academic, and some findings can be uncomfortable for partners. For example, one of my partners was not happy when a research project failed to show significant differences between private and public sector practices. Both sides occasionally failed to clearly articulate expectations.

This tension was sometimes further complicated by frequent changes in decision-making partners' personnel. The person who signed on as a partner on behalf of an organization, with one idea about the nature of the relationship, might be replaced by someone with a quite different view. Governments and other decision-making bodies tend to have a more top-down structure and to change policies more quickly than is the case in universities. Moreover, different partners for the same chair did not necessarily share the same expectations. Yet the chair remained the same person throughout, albeit one who often had to adapt in response to these changes in decision-makers. In my case, I worked with five different directors from one partnership, and the predecessor of each had not had time to explain to our agreement. Such changes and lack of communication limited the decision-making power of new directors and made them hesitant to make new commitments. However, the fact that each chair spans ten years allowed us to build a reputation with our partners that helped overcome some of the strain of transitions. The long-term occupancy also helped to educate partners about differences in and limits on our practices, just as it allowed us to learn how to take those outside the university into account.

There was also tension related to time. On the one hand, our decision-making partners often work under different time constraints that require them to respond quickly and, in turn, to ask for quick responses from us. But for academics, research and capacity-building take longer. There is an inherent tension in these conflicting pressures, a tension that can be exacerbated by the pressure within decision-making organizations for measurable outcomes from the partnership. On the other hand, these partnerships provided us with input from decision-makers on pressing issues where research was needed. They provided avenues for knowledge sharing as well as feedback on research. They offered placements for students who could learn about how to develop and share research relevant to organizations, which often meant that students were in a position to provide the quick responses they needed.

Both sides also learned how to handle all these conflicting pressures. CHSRF has tried to address these tensions in our various meetings with decision-makers and has brought us together on a regular basis. Meeting face to face with a range of decision-makers has done more than offer opportunities to exchange ideas and practices on specific topics; it has also allowed us to address conflicting demands and multiple perspectives. In these meetings, we have increasingly confronted issues of culture differences, such as time frames and approaches to research.

Tensions with Our Universities

As chairs, all but one of us continued to work primarily within a university department and our universities continued to provide us with funding in a variety of forms. In return, our employers expect us to fulfil at least some of our responsibilities as faculty members and to defend the independence of our universities. Here, too, there is opportunity for cultural and other clashes.

One tension relates to teaching and administrative work. While the chair brings prestige to a university, its work takes us out of the classroom. Even though we have not all abandoned teaching regular classes, our loads have been reduced for more than ten years (when sabbaticals are considered). The chair also brings funding for students and support for junior faculty. However, this too can cause tensions. Student funding does not bring teaching money and thus fails to fill the gap we create by leaving the classroom. Our work with our decision-maker partners and with CHSRF frequently takes us away from the university, as do our increasing connections with funding agencies and other governing bodies. This means we often have to limit participation in the administrative work of the university community, which further creates tension with those who take over our teaching and administrative responsibilities.

Another tension relates to the independence of the university. Our absences, and our student funding, can lead to claims that outside funding agencies are taking decision-making roles about issues, such as teaching allocations, out of departments' hands. These issues raise large questions about outside interests entering the university, with a concern that CHSRF priority-setting interfered with university decision-making. Similarly, our work with partners may open us to claims about interference with academic freedom. Would we risk becoming servants rather than critics of external interests? As we pressure universities to recognize and value the work our students do with decision-making partners, we also open up the issue of independence.

CHSRF has helped reduce some of this tension by limiting its requests for reporting and responses from universities. By opening up our spending to support our administrative work, CHSRF has also reduced pressure on university budgets and staff. Perhaps most importantly, it brought in advisors to help negotiate the cultural differences, which led to changes in practices among chairs and between chairs and the organization. These advisors came to our meetings to talk about strategies for getting our kind of work recognized within universities. At the same time, CHSRF came to my university and met with university administrators to talk about the unique features of my chair.

In sum, the chairs' program both expanded and altered the relationships we had to manage. Conflicting cultures and conflicting demands sometimes surfaced. The resources that came with the chair and by the ten-year commitment relieved some of the tension and allowed us to develop practices that balanced the issues for each particular chair. As far as I know, none of us developed a magic solution to these tensions, but we have learned to identify and work with them. Being forewarned can itself be a means of handling these tensions, as can an open discussion of them with partners at an early stage.

Promoting Interdisciplinary Work

As Weingart and Stehr (2000) point out in the preface to their book on interdisciplinary work, the renewed interest in moving beyond disciplinary boundaries comes from the idea that work across disciplines cannot only address large questions in an integrated fashion, but also lead to greater innovation and better science. Health services seem to be particularly appropriate for interdisciplinary work, given the many professions involved and the complexity of the issues raised. The problems can certainly benefit from many minds and many approaches coming together. But as the authors in this edited volume also make clear, interdisciplinary work is difficult. Those in the CHSRF/CIHR chairs program come from a range of disciplines and engage with students from multiple disciplines in an effort to do interdisciplinary work. In this section, I look at some of the challenges, benefits, and lessons from interdisciplinary work.

I have a long history of interdisciplinary work, starting with my master's in Canadian studies many years ago. But such endeavours, in these terms, are about crossing borders among social sciences and the humanities. The disciplines have similar roots and, often, similar methods. Interdisciplinary work in the CHSRF/CIHR chairs programs is more ambitious, and attempts to cross boundaries among social sciences, humanities, and medical sciences. In my view, the biggest source of tension comes not from the quite different paradigms and methods that dominate each field, but rather from the failure to recognize and address these differences. These differences exist not only among these three large categories of research work but also within each of them. We have quite different ways of seeing and doing research. We also have different ways of interacting with colleagues, students, and decision-makers, which often reflect disciplinary practices. We ask different kinds of questions, use different approaches to solve them, seek different kinds of answers, and work with others in a manner that varies enormously from discipline to discipline. Interdisciplinary work is not simply a matter of bringing these many differences together to enrich the whole, because we cannot agree on the shape of the whole unless we recognize and address these differences.

This is much easier to do in theory than in practice. As a social scientist, I have spent time theorizing about paradigms and examining the relationships among theory, method, and the presentation of results. Yet I still struggle with many issues related to working across disciplines and often fail to understand the manner in which others evaluate claims. Two examples highlight critical issues in interdisciplinary work and some lessons for dealing with them.

The first example comes from the students enrolled in the initial intensive course that was part of the Ontario Regional Training Centre's diploma program. York University students were frustrated with what they saw as the dominance of a particular model of evidence in the course. They felt that other approaches were not included or recognized as legitimate ways to approach issues, as would be appropriate in an interdisciplinary setting. They were particularly concerned about truth claims and notions of evidence that were taken more from the medical than the social sciences. In response, and with funding from my chair, they organized a conference with other students in the program and presented papers that offered a broad range of views on evidence and multiple paradigms for approaching health services that challenged old boundaries. The head of CHSRF came and commented in ways that prompted responses as well as addressed them. Together, they explored that benefits and tensions of interdisciplinary work, providing a lesson in how to conduct it.

My second example is from a large, interdisciplinary project titled "Hidden Costs, Invisible Contributions of Unpaid Caregiving." Students and faculty members from the humanities and socials sciences worked together on this interdisciplinary SSHRC-funded project. The project scheduled meetings and workshops that brought people together in creative ways intended to transcend boundaries. But tensions quickly became apparent. It was the students, as well as the external reviewers, who pushed us to confront the different assumptions we each brought to the project – assumptions that grew out of each of our implicit disciplinary approach. As part of this process, the students produced a paper for *Queen's Quarterly* and for a conference on the joys and sorrows of working across disciplines. They were able to progress in building an interdisciplinary research forum after they made their disciplinary assumptions visible to themselves as well as to others. However, it is still often difficult to have journals and peer-review committees accept the methods and approaches of interdisciplinary work.

CHSRF has promoted interdisciplinary work for good reason. Putting the theory into practice, however, requires us to examine our own ways of working in order to figure out how to work with other disciplines. It is also a management issue because it means managing tensions in ways that allow differences to surface and be addressed openly. In spite of CHSRF's efforts, interdisciplinary work in health services is struggling to be recognized and to develop means of recognizing different paradigms as well as different contributions. However, the students, postdoctoral fellows, and junior faculty who have participated in the chairs program are now in a position to advise others, to serve on review panels, and to assess manuscripts that take an interdisciplinary perspective.

Resources

The good news is that CHSRF chairs received ten years of funding, a policy that set us apart from other chairs and faculty members. We had to meet the criteria set out in our proposals, which included experience in handling money, and pass the mandatory midterm review. But we also had some discretion in spending those funds on the projects we had defined in our proposals, albeit under guidance from our governing bodies. We had to be flexible in the allocation of funds in order to be innovative, especially in relation to knowledge exchange, while responding to regulations from our universities and CHSRF, and to the needs of our partners. The bad news is that we had to manage that funding. Not all of us had support in place to do so, and not all of us had processes in place to determine criteria for allocating funds. In addition, conflicts arose between university and CHSRF policies. In this final brief section, I raise some of the issues in money management and offer some lessons I learned in addressing them.

In many universities, new technologies for processing data combined with cutbacks in university funding have meant that the burden of managing money falls increasingly on individual faculty members. There is, however, a qualitative difference in the funding among chairs in this program. For some chairs, their existing projects and university practices meant there was machinery to deal with the financial processes – machinery that took some money management out of their hands. Some chairs also had current programs that had established criteria for funding students, postdoctoral fellows, and junior faculty. But others lacked some or all of these supports.

Moreover, even those chairs who had money management policies and practices in place still had to develop the academic and other criteria for spending on new kinds of projects and practices. Decision-making regarding which projects or people receive funding still requires the chair's involvement, and new issues continually arise. What do you do, for example, when the large chunk of money set aside for a postdoctoral fellowship suddenly becomes available because the person who was awarded the fellowship decided at the last minute to take a faculty position? After this happened to me more than once, I was left with enough money to hire a junior faculty member. My spending allocations also sometimes appeared to contradict university practices related to issues such as rates for travel or legitimate expenditures at meetings, an issue that led to a meeting between my university and CHSRF staff, as well as to formal notification from CHSRF of the different rules that apply.

Support in these money management issues eventually came from three kinds of sources. First, chairs began to share their own strategies for setting criteria to allocate funding and handling money. I was, for instance, able to adapt the procedures for funding graduate students from another chair for my own purposes. Second, advisory boards and partners also shared their experience. For example, another chair suggested that I use my unspent postdoctoral funding to support hiring a junior faculty member, which I did. Third, CHSRF provided advice and approval for spending on administrative personnel. Once I hired someone to manage my money and my time, I became more efficient and effective as a researcher. CHSRF staff also helped explain to the university how and why different rules applied.

The funding allowed chairs not only to support students who learned to work outside the conventional boundaries, but also to pay for exchange activities that would normally be difficult to fund for faculty. The program's flexibility allowed us to support innovative work, pursue innovative exchange, and develop cross-border networks. Reporting and governance requirements, in the end, ensured accountability while encouraging integrative practices and maintaining our academic responsibilities. We learned that there are a variety of ways to manage money, but it must be managed. We learned to look to others for advice on protocols and hire someone to do the actual financial work while retaining the right to make decisions based on academic criteria and the overall purpose of the project.

Conclusion

A year after I took up my chair, I tried to give it back. I tried again a year later. I found the work of managing the experiment overwhelming. It was not for lack of experience in such work: I had chaired a very large department at York University and had been the director of a quite complex school at Carleton, and felt confident in my skills as a manager. However, in those jobs I had an established workplace and a full staff. In the chair, I had neither. Moreover, in those other roles I did not have the same responsibilities to multiple authorities while at the same time seeking to transform aspects of the organization. Equally important, I resisted a focus on managerial work, because I firmly believed I had to be centrally engaged in the research project in order to be an effective mentor and to be knowledgeably involved in exchange.

My political economy perspective led to a concern that as chair in the program I was complicit in the transformation of the university in ways that could threaten academic freedom and curiosity-driven research. The program seemed to fit well with efforts to commercialize university outputs and to reduce accountability to measurement. Our concern with recognizing public intellectuals runs the risk of making us servants of particular publics. For me, the cultural clash I experienced in dealing with CHSRF was an indicator of this risk. In short, I was not sure I wanted to be part of the scaling up from our program to university and community change in this way.

CHSRF staff and some of the others chairs convinced me to stay. So did their willingness to share what they learned from their various leadership styles. For several reasons, I am glad they did. Most importantly, I can see the ways in which chair resources have helped build capacity, especially in creating the supports, space, and connections for students, postdoctoral fellows, and junior faculty to do work that is not only focused on health services, but also linked to practices outside the university. When, for example, the postdoctoral fellows are hired away from my program before their funding is gone, or when I encounter another fellow in a senior decision-making role, I know that at least some parts of the experiment worked. Over the years, these graduates have become resources to me in my work and the chair program. This, in turn, allows me to contribute in other ways to building capacity inside and outside the university. So, for example, when the Centre of Excellence for Women's Health was about to collapse, I had the contacts from my partnership with Health Canada, the flexibility, and the experience necessary to take over, fulfil its commitments to the Bureau of Women's Health and Gender Analysis, and restructure the centre so it could continue without me.

CHSRF staff helped me organize support for the managerial work within the university by providing advice and making their rules more flexible. This is linked to other transformations, both within CHSRF and in our relationship. There has been a cultural shift within CHSRF that is reflected in multiple processes, especially in our reporting mechanism and meeting content. We have openly discussed the risks of becoming too responsive to partners and CHSRF. As a result of sharing experiences and practices with other chairs, I have been able to establish policies and mechanisms for addressing some of my most pressing managerial issues. I have also learned to say no, at least sometimes.

While the above is in many ways a very individual conclusion, there are more general lessons embedded in it. A transformative program like the CHSRF/CIHR chairs program needs to begin by identifying areas of tension and recognizing cultural differences, not only between town and gown, but also among disciplines. It is equally important to acknowledge, from the very beginning, the managerial work involved and to develop mechanisms to deal with it in a manner that respects the centrality of relationships and content to managing within a university and in relation to those outside it. It is also important to explicitly address who the employer is and what rights the funding agencies have to intervene in, and control, everyday practices. Methods of accountability should also be on the agenda. Regular meetings focused on content and sharing expertise among the chairs can promote all of these processes. Good managerial practices are critical and bad ones can critically undermine the overall project of a chair, but they need to be based on a shared understanding of the purpose of the program.

REFERENCES

Beckhard, R. (1969). *Organization development: Strategies and models*. Reading, MA: Addison-Wesley.

Burawoy, M. (2005). 2004 American Sociological Association presidential address: For public sociology. *British Journal of Sociology, 56*(2), 259–94. http://dx.doi.org/10.1111/j.1468-4446.2005.00059.x Medline:15926908

CBC (Canadian Broadcasting Corporation). (1999). *Henry Mintzberg in conversation. Ideas*. Toronto: CBC.

Foucault, M. (1980). *Power/knowledge; selected interviews and other writings, 1972–1977*. New York: Pantheon Books.

Foucault, M. (1997). *Ethics: Subjectivity and truth*. New York: New Press.

Grey, C. (2005). *Critical management studies: Towards a more mature politics*. Paper presented at the Critical Management Studies Conference, Cambridge, England, July 4–6.

Menzies, H. (2005). *No time: Stress and the crisis of modern life*. Vancouver, BC: Douglas and McIntyre.

Mintzberg, H. (1979). *The structuring of organizations*. New York: Prentice-Hall.

Rose, N. (1996). *Inventing our selves*. Cambridge: Cambridge University Press. http://dx.doi.org/10.1017/CBO9780511752179

Smith, D. (1999). *Writing the social critique, theory and investigations*. Toronto: University of Toronto Press.

Stein, J.G. (2001). *The cult of efficiency*. Toronto: Anansi.

Swift, J. (1999). Saving the corporate soul. *Canadian Forum, 78*(June), 16–21.

Turk, J. (2000). *The corporate campus: Commercialization and the dangers to Canada's colleges and universities*. Halifax: James Lorimer & Company.

Weingart, P. & Stehr, N. (Eds.). (2000). *Practicing interdisciplinarity*. Toronto: University of Toronto Press.

11 Evidence-Informed Management in Healthcare Organizations: An Experience in Academic Renewal

JEAN-LOUIS DENIS IN COLLABORATION WITH LISE LAMOTHE AND ANNE MCMANUS

In July 2000, I took on the position of CHSRF/CIHR Chair in Governance and Transformation of Health Care Organizations. The raison d'être of this chair program is to explore the challenges facing, and the strategies supporting, the implementation of evidence-informed management in healthcare organizations.

The chair program has taught us a great deal. In particular, we have learned about the benefits of taking a flexible approach to governing such a program; the fact that knowledge use is a shared responsibility between researchers and practitioners; and that large-scale knowledge exchange activities demand significant financial resources, dedicated staff, and a robust infrastructure. It has also become clear that definite, though semipermeable, boundaries between academic work and managerial roles and practices in healthcare delivery organizations must be maintained, as they help to ensure the generation of research results that benefit both scholars and the organizations being studied.

While the chair program began with a clear plan and accountability framework, it soon gained a life of its own, leading us in directions that we did, and could, not foresee when we began. In order to learn fully from the experiences of the past decade, we have been obliged to consider the dynamic emergence of new issues and perspectives among our partner organizations, as well as the program's own temporal evolution. Furthermore, the specificity of our investigative focus has influenced both our plans and operations.

This chapter is comprised of four sections. Adhering to a process methodology developed in the field of organizational research (Langley & Denis, 2006), in each section we discuss how the chair program relates to challenges confronting applied health services research, capacity building for such research, and knowledge exchange. First, we examine the challenges that face the implementation of evidence-informed management in healthcare organizations. Next, we look at the practice of partnership-based research in general and, specifically, at collaborative research conducted in healthcare organizations. Then, we deal with knowledge exchange activities. In the conclusion, we address a fundamental concern of the chair program: the governance of academic activities in evolving networks. Finally, we share some lessons learned about conducting collaborative applied research and implementing evidence-informed management.

Evidence-Informed Management in Healthcare Organizations

The Complex Nature of Evidence-Informed Management

Scholars increasingly scrutinize the establishment and execution of evidence-informed management in healthcare organizations (Champagne, Lemieux-Charles, & McGuire, 2004; Kovner & Rundall, 2006; Walshe & Rundall, 2001). Programs developed by various funding agencies (e.g., CIHR) and initiatives implemented by healthcare organizations (e.g., knowledge brokers, knowledge networks, communities of practice) are testament to a strong interest in evidence-informed management. The chair program draws on this growing interest to develop and support its various activities.

The field of evidence-based medicine has contributed to the evolution of evidence-informed management. That said, evidence-informed management possesses several unique characteristics that researchers and practitioners cannot ignore. Factors such as those listed below make it a highly complex endeavour (Lomas, Culyer, McCutcheon, McAuley, & Law, 2005; Walshe & Rundall, 2001; Whitley, 1988):

- The need to extract actionable information from a diverse body of evidence (e.g., quantitative and qualitative data, multiple research designs);
- The need to take full account of context and incorporate contextual evidence when designing strategies to increase knowledge use; and
- The relatively loose links between management practices and outcomes.

If the goal is to involve healthcare managers in the use and application of research-based evidence, strategies to promote evidence-informed management must address these issues.

Scholars have identified many of the skills and competencies that managers often rely on when making evidence-informed decisions (Pfeffer & Sutton, 1999; Rousseau, 2006; Rousseau & McCarthy, 2007). Despite the assistance such skills and competencies can provide, evidence-informed management constitutes a clear departure from the dominant managerial culture. Too often, managers rely excessively on authority or consent when making and implementing decisions (Rousseau, 2006). Evidence-informed management, meanwhile, frequently entails significant changes in the way managers conceive of their roles and conduct their relationships with colleagues within and beyond their organizations. At the same time, evidence-informed management promotes the emergence of more flexible leadership structures and styles, and requires that managers have the ability and willingness to debate with their colleagues the actions necessary to achieve the best possible outcomes.

Change also arises in the way various management levels make decisions and develop their roles and functions (Denis, Contandriopoulos, & Beaulieu, 2004). For example, in Canadian healthcare systems, the role of regional health authorities (RHAs) goes beyond planning and control. RHAs typically also support evidence-informed management in healthcare organizations, emphasizing the development of roles that enable organizational and practice-oriented changes. Because evidence-informed management is a significant departure from decision-making norms, it can succeed only in the context of deliberately developed and supported organizational capacities (Denis, Lehoux, & Tré, 2009). It also depends on adapting research processes to promote exchange and debate between researchers and decision-makers (e.g., Cummings, 2003; Denis & Lehoux, 2009; Greenhalgh et al., 2004).

Our Approach to Understanding Evidence-Informed Management

Taking into account all these considerations, the chair program has focused on creating a deeper understanding of the challenges evidence-informed management faces and of the potential of applied health services research to support it. We have based our approach on several assumptions. To begin with, research-based evidence on organizational change and transformation does not take the form of unambiguous prescriptions for decisions and practices. Knowledge that has added value for practitioners must be contextualized, which means that concerned individuals and organizations must have the opportunity to translate abstract knowledge into reasonable hypotheses suitable for their own contexts. The ability to conduct such translation depends, to varying degrees, on organizational capabilities related to individual competencies, information infrastructure, leadership, and the availability of resources for experimentation and innovation (Denis, Lehoux, & Tré, 2009).

Research Partnerships and Evidence-Informed Management

In this section, we discuss the collaborative model of applied research that has emerged since the inception of the chairs program, including its links to the design of experiments that involve a realistic approach to evidence-informed management. We also address the practical experience the chair program has provided to students.

Our Approach to Collaborative Research

We incorporate elements of Mode 1 and Mode 2 scientific research as defined by Gibbons and colleagues (1994). Such research is driven by a cumulative process of knowledge acquisition and is attuned to the importance of both contextualizing and framing enquiries in ways that foster dialogue between researchers and individuals who work in the practice settings studied.

In order to improve our understanding of the transformation and governance of healthcare organizations, we explore several intersecting topics, as follows:

- The collective nature of leadership in complex organizations;
- Strategy-driven change in organizations characterized by distributed expertise and authority;
- The role of managerial functions in inducing change;
- The management of new organizational forms (e.g., networks); and
- The development of new management capabilities.

We have designed our methods so that researchers can track organizational changes over time and discern the influence of governance structure and instruments on the transformative process. Expected outcomes constitute only one factor that sparks organizational change. Therefore, we focus primarily on providing insights for managers (and leading clinicians) on aspects of organizational transformations that appear to be critical for augmenting the benefits of change, whether mandated from outside of the organization or arising from within it.

Our chair program requires and thrives on close linkages with practice settings. As a result, perceived systemic or organizational challenges and dysfunctions are often the triggers that launch our projects. We usually employ a longitudinal case study methodology built on qualitative measures, and track change processes by combining various information sources, such as interviews with key informants, non-participant observations, and secondary data such as meeting minutes and statistics on organizational activities. This approach leads to many face-to-face interactions between researchers and employed staff in the practice settings.

While theoretical lenses and scientific questions guide our inquiries, our explorations can be characterized as collaborative because they rely on the involvement of practitioners, the cooperation of decision-makers, and unfettered access to real-life organizational experiences. Developing close linkages with practice settings influences how we frame our research questions and interpret our findings; at the same time, we take great care not to lose our scientific autonomy. Two of the practical benefits of this collaborative model are the development of interest in evidence-informed management among decision-makers, and the strengthening of our research team's concern for the value our results have for practice settings.

Our research process also supports the promotion of evidence-informed management – but only under certain conditions. In organizational research there is a long tradition of collaborative inquiry: "A deliberate set of interactions and processes designed specifically to bring together those who study social problems and issues (researchers) with those who act on or within those societal problems and issues (decision-makers, practitioners, citizens)" (Denis & Lomas, 2003, S2:1). Recently, together with my colleague Pascale Lehoux, we explored the various styles of collaborative research implemented in order to better understand their implications for the practice of research (Denis & Lehoux, 2009). We discovered a spectrum of collaborative research traditions: from approaches that are essentially driven by problem solving to more participatory or emancipatory approaches that promote self-actualization and empowerment. Since the inception of the chair program, our analysis and experience of collaborative research suggests that a fundamental challenge it faces is the level of control that researchers maintain over the research goals and processes. While the participatory approach regards a high level of researcher control as problematic, we have found that, in contexts where there is a great deal of pressure to conduct collaborative research and where the goal is to implement an evidence-informed agenda, it is critical that researchers take on leadership roles in structuring the investigative process.

One of the primary goals of organizational analysis is the theorization of social processes within organizations and societies (Denis & Lehoux, 2009; Whyte, 1991). To that end, researchers – ourselves included – develop close links with participants in the field while still maintaining relative independence. Striking this balance is essential, especially in a research field that involves partnerships with organizational élites and in which participants often look for instant solutions to their problems or challenges.

The nature of collaborative research requires that we constantly reinforce the distinction between our two roles: that of consultant, which is widespread in healthcare organizations; and that of researcher, who aims to make inquiries without being pressured to respond to immediate demands or demonstrate the instant applicability of research results. In our work, we take academic knowledge as the basis for interactions with practitioners and for reflexive analysis (Schön, 1983). As noted above, we use research-based evidence as a tool to stimulate critical thinking about practices rather than to prescribe specific actions.

In practical applications, most researchers – again, ourselves included – adopt a compromise between the fully participative or collaborative model and the distant or confined model of scientific research (Callon, Lascoumes, & Barthe, 2001). In this hybrid model, each research project is supported by a cooperative agreement with a target organization. Such agreements, which can be thought of as soft contracts between executive teams and researchers, clearly set out organizations' demands and researchers' obligations.

The next step is to use research-based evidence to identify issues that seem to be at the core of management practices – in our case, the business of managing large-scale changes in healthcare organizations. At key moments along this investigative journey, researchers discuss results with concerned practitioners. This process includes three main components:

1. The validation of major interpretive themes with leading informants and practitioners. This element often leads to controversy and enriches our interpretations. It also seems to prompt reflexive thought among practitioners. For example, in one case involving leadership and merger issues, exposure to research-based evidence increased practitioners' sensitivity to the importance of outcomes related to managerial and organizational processes.
2. The identification, in consultation with practitioners, of dilemmas that strongly affect their work and to which research may provide plausible insights (but no absolute solutions). For example, considering ambiguous mandates in healthcare reforms or the instability of political leadership within the healthcare system provides opportunities for collaborative deliberation that involves both researchers and practitioners, a process aimed at identifying innovative practices or potential action levers.
3. The identification of further opportunities for in-depth exploration and the dissemination of our research findings.

Two elements facilitate this model of organizational research in healthcare settings: the circulation of researchers' findings, which helps to generate and sustain a network of researchers and practitioners focused on a given project or issue; and the discussion of research-based evidence around themes that may not, at first sight, be tangible for practicing managers. As an example of the latter, our investigation as of the time of writing focuses on the role of ambiguity in the management of radical restructuring in healthcare organizations. Contrary to many previous studies in the fields of knowledge transfer and evidence-informed management, our work to date reveals that managers are interested in problems and conceptual frames that go beyond their day-to-day challenges.

The chair program's approach to research concurs with CIHR's definition of integrated knowledge transfer; it also aligns with a conceptual approach to knowledge use (Denis, Lehoux, & Champagne, 2004). Furthermore, it helps to preserve the specificities and potential added value of scholarly work, while creating opportunities for mutual learning between researchers and practitioners. By maintaining strict control over the research process, we believe that we are able to preserve investigative autonomy while still learning a great deal from the practice settings we explore. It is probably also true that this clear delineation of roles and responsibilities better positions decision-makers to learn from our research. In the event, however, that a group of decision-makers reacts too strongly to our research findings, our protocols call for the suspension of the collaboration. In our experience, this has happened only once, and we suspect that our efforts – early in each relationship – to reduce expectations regarding the immediate utility of our research findings minimize the risk of collaborative dysfunction and in fact foster dialogue around broader issues and concerns.

While collaborative research is a plausible way to increase the use of research-based evidence, it is vital to ensure that the knowledge produced is not manipulative (Argyris & Schön, 1989) or biased. This is especially crucial in situations where research mainly involves the practices of organizational élites. Our experience suggests that collaborations need to be coupled with a constant assertion of the independence of researchers' viewpoints and a high tolerance – within research teams and practice settings alike – for competing interpretations of organizational processes and the operational implications of research. When this occurs, collaborative interactions are sufficient to clarify, for researchers and decision-makers, the distinctions between scholarly and managerial roles and objectives.

An R&D Approach to Collaborative Research

Another way of framing collaborative research is to conceive of it as a research-and-development (R&D) operation in the field of social inquiry. While relatively underdeveloped in social and organizational research, the R&D approach is somewhat similar to the problem-solving approach associated with knowledge use in organizations (Denis, Lehoux, & Champagne, 2004). The work we undertook on the development of a governance framework and standards for Accreditation Canada offers a good example of R&D-style collaboration (Denis, Champagne, Pomey, Préval, & Tré, 2005). In that case, Accreditation Canada used our research team's initial governance framework to establish a consulting process with senior executives and board members across the country. After the organization validated the framework, we used a similar process to develop corresponding standards for accreditation purposes.

While an R&D approach to collaborative research appears to have great potential for transforming knowledge into action, it entails a different type of relationship between researchers and decision-makers. This is because collaborative research is, by nature, contractual, and because the frameworks and standards we produce as researchers become resources for our partner organizations. Those organizations can use and transform our research products as they wish to serve their own main missions. The knowledge use promoted in the R&D approach is, therefore, much more instrumental for decision-makers than the conceptual process described earlier.

Graduate Student Training

One of the chair program's objectives is to develop capacity in health services research. To that end, we have actively involved graduate students and postdoctoral fellows in all our projects. From 2000 to the time of writing, sixty-three students have been associated with our program and it has provided financial support (e.g., scholarships, conference travel funding) for thirty-nine of them.

Fieldwork has brought many of our students into contact with researchers located outside the University of Montreal, our home institution. For others, involvement in the field has allowed them to test the core tenets of their doctoral theses with decision-makers and to gather critical information from practice settings. Fieldwork is also an occasion for our students to get actively involved in knowledge exchange activities. The only potential drawback is that some students find it difficult to balance their academic responsibilities with their involvement in practice settings. This issue becomes particularly acute when students still have courses to complete. In my experience, the best way for students to strike a healthy balance is to maintain regular contact with their research directors.

Knowledge Exchange Activities that Support Evidence-Informed Management

The Forum Series

As part of the chair program, we initiated activities that aimed to stimulate linkages and exchanges with, and knowledge use in, healthcare practice settings. One of our first tasks was the 2003 launch of our Forum series, which convenes four times a year. We hoped these gatherings would offer a neutral space in which the main objective would be to discuss different viewpoints on managerial situations without focusing on specific local contexts and issues unless doing so could shed light on broader issues. Research-based evidence is but one component of Forum sessions; the main focus is on researchers' and practitioners' experiences, rather than on formal presentations of research findings.

Forum sessions have enabled us to broaden our network of decision-makers by bringing together healthcare managers who come from a variety of organizations and decision-making and governance levels, and who are not necessarily involved directly in our research endeavours. A fundamental Forum rule is that these individuals participate not as representatives of their specific institutions, but as people willing to share practical knowledge and experience. While researchers participate in the Forum, they do not constitute a majority. We also invite graduate students to attend sessions with the expectation they will learn about the challenges healthcare organizations face and the processes by which research-based evidence can be made meaningful for practitioners. In addition, the meetings allow students and researchers to identify research gaps and to learn about how best to frame research problems and processes in order to inform managerial practices.

We select Forum participants not only according to their job profiles, but also with an eye to their interest in taking part in open exchanges and their ability to adhere to the rules that guide our discussions. These rules are very simple: decision-makers must agree to keep the content of Forum sessions confidential, to respect the right of all participants to voice their opinions, and to not promote their own agendas. This last point is crucial because, as noted earlier, Forum participants are drawn from various governance levels and some attendees are in competition with each other.

At the end of each session, we synthesize the key points discussed and propose further avenues of exploration. Some of the themes that have been addressed since the launch of the Forum series include network management, population health strategies for healthcare organizations, and incentives for change and improvement. An analysis of the first three years of the Forum experience (2003 to 2005) has been published in *Infolettre*, the chair program's newsletter. We intend to build on this analysis in order to assess further the potential and limitations of such an activity to integrate research-based evidence in healthcare management. One possibility is to develop practice guidelines for healthcare managers founded on research-based evidence and the integration of experiential knowledge. Managing networks in healthcare organizations would be a suitable topic for developing such guidelines.

The Forum's structure is most strongly informed by the enlightenment model of knowledge use (Denis, Lehoux, & Champagne, 2004). The sessions create loose networks by drawing the worlds of research and practice closer together. In turn, the circulation of ideas throughout these networks increases awareness of the potential of research to inform managerial practices. Following their participation in the Forum, practitioners return to their organizations with insights and ideas that hold the potential to influence how they frame problems and solutions. While researchers are not directly involved in translating Forum-derived insights into specific management practices, the gatherings often trigger further exchange and collaboration between researchers and decision-makers.

The Forum also entails a strategic model of knowledge use, which guides the definition of the themes discussed at each session. Managers come to these events when they believe they can learn something that could help them confront their emergent issues. They do not necessarily look for solutions, but for innovative perspectives; their interest in knowledge is, therefore, contingent on their real-world organizational challenges. This strategic model of knowledge use differs from the one we use in our program of applied health services research (discussed earlier), where we place less value on immediate utility.

Broadly speaking, our experience of hosting Forum sessions suggests that managers and decision-makers want to discuss abstract ideas and concepts, as long as they can relate them to concrete processes and problems in their organizations. Practitioners' various interests make it occasionally difficult to secure a stable group of participants. From what we have observed to date, however, group stability from session to session is likely to lead to increased learning.

As of the time of writing, we have been only partly successful in securing the attendance of a core group of participants. The positive side of participants' diversity is that it might contribute to the diffusion of ideas across a broader network of organizations.

The Forum sessions also help to develop other types of linkages between, and joint activities among, researchers and practice settings. For example, in 2005 we convened a session to address contract management in healthcare organizations. The material we developed for, and during, this event provided the basis for further research with the Association of Health Care Organizations in Quebec (AQESSS), and for a meeting on the topic with the chief executive officers of Quebec's regional health authorities and the deputy minister of the province's Ministry of Health and Social Services.

In order to improve the relevance of the themes discussed at the Forum sessions, to increase the stability of attendees' participation, and to enlarge our operations, we developed close partnerships with key practitioners in the field, and with the Institut national de santé publique du Québec (INSPQ). Through our collaboration with the INSPQ, the Forum became more institutionalized and now has an official program that sets out annual activities in Montreal and Quebec City (INSPQ's two sites of operation). This collaboration also enlarged our network of researchers. Academic colleagues from the National School for Public Administration (ENAP) and Laval University facilitate the Quebec City sessions, and this partnership has significantly increased the penetration of the Forum's activities in practice settings.

Seminar Series: Knowledge and Practice Change in Healthcare Organizations

In order to stimulate wider engagement with the topic of knowledge use through the chair program, Dr Lehoux and I developed a seminar series focusing on knowledge and practice change in healthcare organizations. Offered five times since 2001, this interdisciplinary seminar brings together multiple perspectives on knowledge use in clinical, organizational, and policy settings. It also enables participants to develop a knowledge management strategy for healthcare agencies based on the external-consultant model. The seminar series deliberately mixes graduate students and field practitioners who are interested in the contributions research-based evidence might make to their organizations.

One of our main challenges has been to balance theoretical analysis with practitioners' interest in tangible knowledge-management tools and methods. We continue to struggle with this issue, but we believe it is valuable to maintain a tension between conceptual development and instrumental application. We also believe that, by exploiting this tension, participants can develop innovative approaches to knowledge use in their organizations.

Our overall experience of running the Forum series suggests there is strong demand for learning opportunities that bring academics, graduate students, postdoctoral fellows, and practitioners together to debate the evolution of knowledge transfer. For students who wish to develop careers in applied health services research, the question of knowledge use and how to promote the appropriate application of research-based evidence is critical. In addition, my long-term involvement in CHSRF's Executive Training for Research Application (EXTRA) program has allowed me to expand the chair' s education activities to a wider spectrum of healthcare managers and decision-makers across Canada (Denis, Lomas, & Stipich, 2008).

The Chair Program's Newsletter

The publication of *Infolettre*, the chair program's quarterly electronic newsletter focusing on managerial and evaluation practices in healthcare, involves a broad network of academics and mobilizes students and practitioners. Each issue has three main components:

- A *thema*, which summarizes a topic (based on the current Forum topic) in healthcare management;
- A viewpoint prepared by a practitioner on the *thema*; and
- An article written for practitioners and related to the field of evaluation in health services and health promotion practices.

Infolettre is published in both French and English, and we distribute it to more than 750 people employed in the healthcare management field. We see *Infolettre* as a way to increase public awareness, beyond Forum participants, of the potential contributions of research to management, and to showcase investigations that may be of relevance to managers. While it is difficult at this stage to assess *Infolettre*'s impact, feedback from readers leads us to believe the newsletter is a valuable complement to the Forum, and that it has helped to increase our program's impact across many settings and for a diverse audience.

Systematization and Alliances

Our knowledge exchange efforts to date strongly suggest that systematic processes and formal alliances foster close and beneficial connections between researchers and practitioners, as well as between research-based evidence and practice settings. Collaboration with healthcare managers and INSPQ has become a key component of the chair program's governance model. Along the way, we have come to realize that this model ought to derive from activities and should not involve setting up a priori structures. However, establishing and implementing linkages and exchange activities requires a formal governance structure as well as personnel responsible for coordinating tasks, relations with practice settings, and diffusion activities. Resources provided by the chair program are essential for supporting these components.

Impact on Evidence-Based Management

While we feel positive about the chair program's initiatives, it is clear that their impact on the implementation of evidence-based management in healthcare organizations is indirect. The development of interest in, and the ability to use, research-based evidence to support change and continuous improvement largely depends on an organization's internal processes. Our work does not act directly on those processes. Nevertheless, we firmly believe that it creates positive contexts that increase decision-makers' determination to look to research and researchers for insights into how best to deal with problems and strategic issues. Our work also supports the development, within our own scholarly community, of greater concern for our responsibility to promote the use of research-based evidence.

Concluding Remarks

Issues of Governance

Traditionally, governance has been conceived of as the responsibility of a formal authoritative body (e.g., the board of directors of a corporation). In this formulation, it is concerned with accountability issues and the control of key organizational members, such as chief executive officers and other senior executives (Davis, Schoorman, & Donaldson, 1997). This view on governance has been criticized for being out of touch with the challenges contemporary organizations face and the level of cooperation required to deal with complex social problems and respond to demands for innovation.

For our chair program, we have taken a flexible approach to governance. This approach has proven ideal for governing loose networks of individuals and organizations, and has enabled us to implement and monitor innovative projects and methods of solving social and organizational problems. Flexible governance emphasizes the role of emergent opportunities and enables greater participation in networks and partnerships that resonate with sundry program components. We do not govern the chair program; rather, we participate in the development of governance capacities that aim to expand program activities and opportunities. Taking a flexible approach also makes sense in light of the fact that chairs are relatively fragile entities: their resource bases are modest and CHSRF support has a scheduled end. Flexible governance has enabled us to make the most of the program's financial and time constraints.

In 2001, we formalized the chair program's governance structure by establishing an advisory board. This group comprised academics from the University of Montreal; external partners, such as RHA CEOs; and civil servants known for their experience with the types of activities we planned. The advisory board helped us to determine the chair program's broad orientation during our initial stage of development. It also provided suggestions for innovative activities and advice on how to connect our program with practitioners in the field.

We eventually revised our governance structure as a result of changes to the professional roles of some advisory board members; the program's natural evolution; and CHSRF's monitoring of our progress through our annual reports, accountability framework, and renewal process. This second-generation structure is less formal and is based on partnerships across the healthcare sector. Two principles underlie our new governance model: the importance of valuing strategic alliances with key stakeholders in the field; and the importance of targeting dominant partners who will also contribute to the scale of our operations through their expertise and financial or in-kind support. Adhering to these principles, we have developed close alliances with a wide variety of healthcare sector stakeholders. Our current arrangements are designed to develop and sustain such collaborations.

The chair program's governance experience also illustrates the importance of research initiatives in implementing new partnerships. At the same time, our flexible approach to governance seems better adapted to, and more effective at, gaining external support. In 2008, for example, CIHR approved our team grant proposal on health system reconfiguration. This funding will support research partnerships, graduate student training, and knowledge exchange activities for five years (2008 to 2013), and represents a major investment that will help to sustain the chair program after 2010, the official sunset date of CHSRF's financial support. In preparing the grant application, our team benefited from strategic alliances with external stakeholders that provided opportunities for research and knowledge exchange activities. While the team grant is a natural evolution of the chair program, it will have its own advisory committee composed both of researchers and field practitioners.

Supporting Evidence-Informed Management and Research Partnerships

The chair program has taught us important lessons about evidence-informed management in healthcare organizations and systems. We have also learned a great deal about how best to conduct collaborative applied research.

Evidence-informed management is a priority for many healthcare executives and organizations. It arises from the need to contextualize knowledge, and follows, as noted earlier, an enlightenment model of knowledge use, whereby research-based evidence enriches the framing of problems and solutions in organizations and systems. The downside of this model is that it often demands a great deal of time from researchers and practitioners because it is largely based on face-to-face interactions. In our experience, partnerships with external agencies have empowered the chair's program to grow operations – for example, the scale of our consultative encounters with practitioners – and ensure they are relevant to the real-world issues that affect healthcare organizations.

These collaborative alliances present significant opportunities for engaging in innovative investigations, knowledge exchange activities, and training graduate students and postdoctoral fellows. The benefits from such partnerships, however, depend on researchers' capacity to maintain scientific autonomy, and researchers' and practitioner' ability to tolerate controversy over the meaning and implications of research findings. While graduate students and postdoctoral fellows may gain a great deal from participating in research partnerships (e.g., knowledge of practice settings, input from practitioners in the formulation of their problem and interpretation of research findings), their academic supervisors nevertheless must pay careful attention in order to guarantee a strong scholarly anchor throughout their studies.

Final Thoughts

The chair program has enabled a deep and thorough exploration of the challenges facing evidence-informed management in healthcare organizations. It has enriched our understanding of both the potential and limitations of various approaches to support the use of research-based evidence in organizations and systems, and has helped us develop a realistic approach to advance evidence-informed management. We now understand much more clearly what we, as academic researchers, can do to encourage the uptake and application of research-based evidence and to involve students in this vital facet of health services research. As an experiment in academic renewal, the chair program also illuminates the benefits of flexible governance when undertaking collaborative applied research with a network of external partners.

REFERENCES

Argyris, C., & Schön, D.A. (1989). Participatory action research and action science compared: A commentary. *American Behavioral Scientist, 32*(5), 612–23. http://dx.doi.org/10.1177/0002764289032005008

Callon, M., Lascoumes, P., & Barthe, Y. (2001). *Agir dans un monde incertain: Essai sur la démocratie technique*. Paris: Seuil.

Champagne, F., Lemieux-Charles, L., & McGuire, W. (2004). Introduction: Towards a broader understanding of the use of knowledge and evidence in health care. In L. Lemieux-Charles & F. Champagne (Eds.), *Using knowledge and evidence in health care* (pp. 3–17). Toronto: University of Toronto Press.

Cummings, J. (2003). *Knowledge sharing: A review of the literature*. Operations Evaluation Department Working Papers. Washington, DC: World Bank.

Davis, J.H., Schoorman, F., & Donaldson, L. (1997). Toward a stewardship theory of management. *Academy of Management Review, 22*(1), 20–47.

Denis, J.-L., Champagne, F., Pomey, M.-P., Préval, J., & Tré, G. (2005). *Toward a framework for the analysis of governance in health care organizations and systems. Preliminary report presented to the Canadian Council on Health Services Accreditation*. Montreal: CCHSA.

Denis, J.-L., Contandriopoulos, D., & Beaulieu, M.-D. (2004). Regionalization in Canada: A promising heritage to build on. *Healthcare Papers, 5*(1), 40–5, discussion 96–9. Medline:15496814

Denis, J.-L., & Lehoux, P. (2009). Collaborative research: Renewing action and governing science. In D.A. Buchanan & A. Bryman (Eds.), *The Sage handbook of organizational research methods* (pp. 363–80). Thousand Oaks, CA: Sage.

Denis, J.-L., Lehoux, P., & Champagne, F. (2004). Knowledge utilization on fine-tuning dissemination and contextualizing knowledge. In L. Lemieux-Charles & F. Champagne (Eds.), *Using knowledge and evidence in health care: Multidisciplinary perspectives* (pp. 18–40). Toronto: University of Toronto Press.

Denis, J.-L., Lehoux, P., & Tré, G. (2009). L'utilisation des connaissances produites. In V. Ridde & C. Dagenais (Eds.), *Approches et pratiques en évaluation de programme* (pp. 177–91). Montreal: Les Presses de l'Université de Montréal.

Denis, J.-L., & Lomas, J. (2003). Convergent evolution: The academic and policy roots of collaborative research. *Journal of Health Services Research & Policy, 8*(Suppl 2), 1–6. http://dx.doi.org/10.1258/135581903322405108 Medline:14596741

Denis, J.-L., Lomas, J., & Stipich, N. (2008). Creating receptor capacity for research in the health system: The Executive Training for Research Application (EXTRA) program in Canada. *Journal of Health Services Research & Policy, 13*(Suppl 1), 1–7. http://dx.doi.org/10.1258/jhsrp.2007.007123 Medline:18325161

Gibbons, M., Limoges, C., Nowotny, H., Schwartzman, S., Scott, P., & Trow, M. (1994). *The new production of knowledge: The dynamics of science and research in contemporary societies*. London: Sage.

Greenhalgh, T., Robert, G., Bates, P., Kyriakidou, O., Macfarlane, F., & Peacock, R. (2004). *How to spread good ideas: A systematic review of the literature on diffusion, dissemination and sustainability of innovations in health service delivery and organization. Report for the NCCSDO*. London: London School of Hygiene and Tropical Medicine.

Kovner, A.R., & Rundall, T.G. (2006). The promise of evidence-based management. *Frontiers of Health Services Management, 22*(3), 3–22. Medline:16604900

Langley, A., & Denis, J.-L. (2006). Neglected dimensions of organizational change: Towards a situated view. In R. Lines, I.G. Stensaker, & A. Langley (Eds.), *New perspectives on organizational change and learning* (pp. 136–61). Bergen, Norway: Fagbokforlaget.

Lomas, J., Culyer, T., McCutcheon, C., McAuley, L., & Law, S. (2005). *Conceptualizing and combining evidence for health system guidance (final report)*. Ottawa: Canadian Health Services Research Foundation.

Pfeffer, J., & Sutton, R.I. (1999). *The knowing-doing gap: How smart companies turn knowledge into action*. Cambridge, MA: Harvard Business School Press.

Rousseau, D.M. (2006). Is there such a thing as "evidence-based management"? *Academy of Management Review, 31*(2), 256–69. http://dx.doi.org/10.5465/AMR.2006.20208679

Rousseau, D.M., & McCarthy, S. (2007). Educating managers from an evidence-based perspective. *Academy of Management Learning & Education, 6*(1), 84–101. http://dx.doi.org/10.5465/AMLE.2007.24401705

Schön, D.A. (1983). *The reflective practitioner: How professionals think in action*. New York: Basic Books.

Walshe, K., & Rundall, T.G. (2001). Evidence-based management: From theory to practice in health care. *The Milbank Quarterly, 79*(3), 429–57, IV–V. http://dx.doi.org/10.1111/1468-0009.00214 Medline:11565163

Whyte, W.F. (1991). *Social theory for action: How individuals and organizations learn to change.* Newbury Park, CA: Sage.

Whitley, R. (1988). The management sciences and managerial skills. *Organization Studies, 9*(1), 47–68. http://dx.doi.org/10.1177/017084068800900110

12 A Home Away from Home: The Influence of Organizational Setting on One Chair's Program

PAULA GOERING

From the beginning, the CHSRF/CIHR chairs program emphasized the need for contributions from each chair's home institution. The application process required a description of the institution and the supports it had to offer. This support was monitored as part of an annual reporting process and, in the early days, was sometimes insufficient, especially in terms of space requirements and administrative assistance. The planners had assumed that the chairs would be employees of university departments and would need protected time to fulfil the functions of their new positions. I was the only chair not employed by a university and was instead the leader and manager of a health services research unit in a psychiatric hospital. My experience regarding home institution support was uniformly positive. This raises a question about whether there was a particularly good fit between what the program was trying to accomplish and the atypical organizational setting. There has been some discussion in the literature about knowledge production that suggests this might be the case.

The wider literature on changes in the roles of universities includes frequent reference to the ideas of Gibbons and colleagues (1994), who delineate two archetypal models of knowledge production that they refer to as Mode 1 and Mode 2. Mode 1 is a traditional model of academia in which the creation of knowledge occurs within disciplines, and the control of both the research agenda and also quality assessment lies firmly within the hands of the academic community. Mode 2 sees the creation of knowledge as an interactive process that includes multidisciplinary teams and is firmly linked to application. Many of Mode 2's attributes, such as collaboration and close connections between theoretical and practical work, are highly compatible with the philosophy and programs of the chairs program. The postulated shift in higher education from Mode 1 to Mode 2 includes the creation of new contexts for knowledge production and exchange (Denis, Lehoux, & Champagne, 2004). Mode 2 also involves more diverse research settings, such that universities are no longer the sole sources of new knowledge (Gibbons et al., 1994). Theorists suggest that advantages of the socially distributed model of knowledge production include the ability to be more strategic and flexible in implementing innovations, but the current literature has not explored this idea.

Ferlie and Wood (2003) examine a number of health services research units in the United Kingdom using the Mode 1 and Mode 2 conceptual frameworks as their lens. They find that aspects of the ideal Mode 2 environment, as defined by Pettigrew (cited in Ferlie & Wood, 2003), were present in most but not all of the units. A cardiovascular research unit in a teaching hospital operated very much like a traditional academic setting, illustrating that institutional location alone does not define the characteristics of an organizational setting. Across the other settings, they find instances where research problems were framed in the context of application and where diffusion occurred in the context of production; typically there were heterogeneous research teams, and social and political accountability were generally high. They also find a mix of Mode 1 and Mode 2 output indicators, and note that the traditional measures of peer-reviewed grants, publications, and knowledge base contributions retained considerable power alongside measures of uptake and impact such as liaison with users, improvements in clinical services, incorporation of results into policy guidelines, and exchange and collaboration. These findings agree with the belief that, rather than a full shift away from it, we need to retain some of the principles and practices associated with Mode 1, while valuing knowledge use and the intense relationships between researchers and users that are associated with Mode 2 (Denis et al., 2004). A hybrid model may be the more realistic and preferred option.

One interesting finding from these case studies was the powerful influence external funding had on research work (Ferlie & Wood, 2003). A diversification in the funding sources, beyond peer-reviewed granting agencies, clearly influenced the research question, the structure of relationships with external parties, and career paths. Mode 2 has been stimulated by what Denis and colleagues (2004) refer to as the new entrepreneurship in research, where academics are involved in the management of various kinds of revenue-generating research units. We will return to this idea in our discussion of the chair's program.

It is timely to look more closely and critically at the effect of organizational setting on research production and translation. Within Canada, there has been a lively ongoing debate about whether new applied chair programs should be designed to prefer, or even require, placement outside of universities. As CIHR adopted the CHSRF/CIHR chairs program funding model for a new set of applied health services chairs, CHSRF asked that placement in a non-university setting be a condition of funding for one specific program that had applied for a chair award. CHSRF's board of trustees also discussed whether service organizations should administer its research programs. Some authors believe that we should train a new generation of researchers, many of whom will occupy positions within the healthcare system rather than within university departments (Mitton & Bate, 2007). Others delineate the advantages and disadvantages of this research model (Chafe & Dobrow, 2008). Debates and discussions about these changes in practice should be informed by the lessons from the natural experiment of the CHSRF/CIHR chairs program.

In this chapter I argue that locating one chair's program in a non-university setting was successful, and the interaction of the program and various organizational factors resulted in several clear benefits. The location also created or amplified tensions that needed to be recognized and managed in order to maximize the unique opportunities associated with such knowledge production environments.

The Characteristics of the Organizational Setting

As is often the case, there were multiple components to the organizational setting. There were two "home institutions" for this chair that had a major influence on how its program was implemented. The first home was the Health Systems Research and Consulting Unit (HSRCU) at the Centre for Addiction and Mental Health (CAMH). The second was the University of Toronto's Department of Psychiatry, where most HSRCU scientists had a primary, status-only appointment and where I am a full professor and at the time held a senior executive position. A brief description of each of these organizations, at the time when the chair was awarded in 2001, follows.

The HSRCU, which no longer exists in the same form, was a multidisciplinary team of seven scientists, thirteen support and administrative staff, and several affiliated consultants working under my leadership since 1990. Its mandate was to promote the use of scientific information to develop an integrated, accessible, and cost-effective system to deliver addictions and mental health services in Ontario, and to produce knowledge useful in the development of best practices and the ongoing improvement of policies, program, and systems. Fulfilling this mandate entailed four complementary domains of work: health services and systems research, program/system evaluation and monitoring, education, and consultation. The unit had well-developed partnerships with provincial and federal mental health policy groups. Funding for the HSRCU came from a mix of sources. A core budget from CAMH provided salary support for all of the scientists and two of the administrative staff. An equivalent amount of external funding from research and consulting activities was used to employ the remainder of the support staff and cover other educational and travel expenses. The HSRCU was one of the largest of five research units among the Social, Prevention, and Health Policy Research Department at CAMH.

CAMH is the largest mental health and addictions facility in Canada and has been designated a centre of excellence by the World Health Organization (WHO). It operates central clinical and research facilities in Toronto, Ontario, as well as satellite education and community development offices across the province. While the centre's work focuses on the needs of Ontario communities, its impact extends nationally and internationally. CAMH's communications, marketing, and educational resources, combined with a province-wide network, work together to ensure rapid dissemination and testing of best practices in the field.

HSRCU was also a centre for excellence for the University of Toronto's Department of Psychiatry's health systems program, which had thirteen other programs that provided leadership and coordination across a network of seventeen affiliated teaching hospitals. The department of psychiatry is one of the largest in the world and has over 700 faculty members, 30 per cent of whom are engaged in full-time academic activities. As a group, these academics are very interdisciplinary; about one third are not physicians, and many come from other professional and social science backgrounds. Each faculty member has a home within one of the programs, and at that time there were ten that were clinically based and four – including the health systems program – that cut across the clinical domains. I co-led this program and was vice chair of programs and planning for the department.

My application for a chair award was entitled "Generating and Disseminating Best Practices in Mental Health." I devised it with input from HSRCU staff and deliberately aligned it with the mission and mandates of both home institutions. Plans included a number of activities such as:

- Hiring a knowledge broker, co-funded by the decision-making partner at the Mental Health Rehabilitation and Reform Branch (MHRRB) of the Ministry of Health and Long-Term Care (MOHLTC);
- Recruiting another social scientist with expertise in qualitative methods to increase research and training capacity;
- Implementing a summer studentship program for undergraduate and master's students;
- Increasing the supervision of graduate students and fellows; and
- Continuing research and consulting activities through the establishment of closer relationships with the provincial and national partners.

The primary decision-making partner, MHRRB, was actively involved with the HSRCU prior to the chair's award through a series of policy-relevant research projects that they had conducted over a number of years (Wasylenki & Goering, 1995). This relationship was formalized as a result of the chair award, and linkage and exchange between the two intensified (Goering, Butterill, Jacobson, & Sturtevant, 2003).

This organizational setting is a complex one, with many reporting relationships. Although the HSRCU was embedded within a service delivery agency, it was not located in the decision-making partner's policy environment (other than through the jointly funded knowledge broker position who, for a time, had a part-time office there). It was outside of the university in the sense that the chair and all of the scientists and staff were employees of the hospital that provided its budget. The close ties I maintained with the department of psychiatry kept the program connected to the university through a medical school department, which has a somewhat different academic culture and administration than cognate departments. The HSRCU was thus not a pure Mode 2 or embedded research model, which may not exist except as a theoretical ideal, but rather a hybrid version that shares many of the characteristics of applied research units situated within universities.

Organizational Factors that Facilitated the Implementation of the Chair's Program

In a previous paper, I identify several factors in university environments that can hinder and/or help the practice of knowledge translation (Jacobson, Butterill, & Goering, 2004). The same factors are relevant to embedded research environments located outside of the university. Four of these factors – structure, orientation, incentives/promotion, and available resources and support – came into play at various times as the chair's program was implemented.

The structure of HSRCU was conducive in many ways to the execution of the chair's program, in that I, as its senior manager, could leverage a platform of resources to meet the program's aims. I did not have to build from scratch, but could focus on renovating an existing structure with an already-strong foundation. HSRCU included scientists who had a considerable amount of protected time for research, since they did not have the usual university faculty commitment to course work and teaching. They were, however, open to becoming more involved in knowledge exchange and training. I introduced a new knowledge broker position, which allowed for increased exchanges with outside organizations, similar to adding more doors and windows to an existing structure. There had never been such a position within the hospital, so I had to define and negotiate a new job description and classification with human resources. I was able to define the role at the manager level so that I could recruit a senior individual highly skilled in organizational change. As I have described in published reports (Goering et al., 2003; Dewa, Butterill, Durbin, & Goering, 2004), this person played a key role in the chair's ability to conduct research using an interactive knowledge translation model. It took considerable flexibility and willingness to experiment by the home institutions' administrative offices for this to happen. Although knowledge brokers are sometimes situated within universities, a 2006 survey revealed that 70 per cent of them were based in other organizations (Lomas, 2007). This, and my experience, suggests it may be easier to introduce and support untested roles in less conservative institutional cultures.

Over time, the knowledge broker became an ambassador for the chair's research within CAMH, as she participated in planning exercises with clinical managers and organized educational forums that included both researchers and providers. This gave us both an expanded platform on which to present and enact the linkage and exchange functions of the chair's program, and also greater currency and visibility for knowledge translation activities within the larger research department.

The orientations of a hospital and of a medical school department are naturally sympathetic to applied research, since practice and service are intrinsic to their mandates. As Denis and colleagues (2004) point out, Mode 2 research fits quite naturally with the process of clinical and health services research, which aims to move rapidly from the creation to application of new knowledge. The consulting practice within the HSRCU drew upon this practice/service orientation to give support and credibility to its activities. Our new social scientist conducted qualitative research that helped us to better understand how interdisciplinary teams that include experienced clinicians and administrators use consulting as a means of knowledge transfer (Jacobson, Butterill, & Goering, 2005). A certain degree of authority and trust was also conferred on the consultants through their membership in CAMH and the university (Jacobson & Goering, 2006).

Mode 1 continues to wield significant defensive power in regard to the use of performance indicators as incentives for researchers (Ferlie & Wood, 2003). Although few would argue that recognition through the traditional use of peer-reviewed publications and grants should be eliminated or is wholly unimportant (Landry, 2007), the challenge is to gain official recognition for the time-consuming activities that are associated with applied research and knowledge transfer. Two systems within the chair's program setting reward scientists: the university, where promotion panels adjudicate movement through the ranks; and the hospital, where supervisors are responsible for annual performance reviews. There was some progress in modifying traditional academic criteria in both systems.

Within the department of psychiatry, I, as a senior member, was able to introduce and support the implementation of a revised definition of one of the existing categories within the promotion policy. I altered the definition of creative professional activity to include impact on services and policy. I also modified the definitions of documentation and procedures and, during my time a chair, acted as a champion for these changes by sitting on the promotions committee and providing advice to those preparing their applications using new criteria.

This successful change, which has been profiled nationally (CHSRF, 2006), was probably easier to make in a medical school department where the decision-making structure in regards to promotion procedures does not include the issue of tenure or negotiations with a faculty association. When CAMH began to develop its own process and procedures for scientist promotion, I was asked to participate. Knowledge about broadening the measurement of academic performance was thus transferred from the University of Toronto to the teaching hospital.

The availability of resources and supports played a major role in the expansion of our teaching and supervision capacity. In a university environment, it is unusual for consulting to be viewed as the activity of an organization rather than an individual faculty member. Without the pooled profits from our HSRCU consulting practice, we would have been unable to offer a summer student program, which worked to enrich our teaching activities, expose students to health services research in mental health and addictions, and allowed them to decide whether to pursue further studies. Shortly after the chair was created, the chief executive officer of CAMH, who was a member of the chair's advisory committee, realized that the allocation of external funds did not include an important component – stipends for fellows. He arranged for the CAMH Foundation to set up a fund that would allow us to recruit and support one fellow for the duration of the chair. It was as if he had given the chair's program a ten-year line of credit, which led to more latitude to use our resources to advance the aims of the program.

Problems and Tensions Created or Amplified by a Non-University Setting

Those who are interested in the possible benefits of embedded research and training sites should not lose sight of what can be lost by moving out of the university. Teaching responsibilities, other than continuing medical education, are not typically a major part of scientists' job descriptions in non-university settings. Although they may have more time for research and knowledge transfer, they may lose the intellectual stimulation associated with classroom and seminar education. They will also have to make a special effort in order to gain access to students for supervision as research trainees. The chair's program encouraged cross-appointments and developed new graduate courses as strategies to alleviate these limitations. Doing so required negotiating mutual responsibilities and benefits, as well as making adjustments to accommodate different organizational contexts.

Working with other colleagues, I initiated a plan to teach a graduate course within the university's health policy management and evaluation department. As I did so, my ideas focused on the use of consulting as a means of knowledge transfer. Though my proposal stated that I would volunteer unpaid faculty time, the department made a guarded response to my offer. It noted that my course outline was too focused on practice and did not have enough theoretical and research methods to qualify as a graduate course. I developed a more general course on knowledge transfer and exchange that included more conceptual and methodological content. Preparing and teaching this course proved to be a stimulating intellectual exercise that expanded my knowledge. At the same time, the inclusion of practitioners (such as government policy advisors, consultants, and knowledge brokers) as guest speakers was consistently appreciated by the students, who commented on the usefulness of the knowledge for their future careers.

Academic freedom and the safeguards needed to protect it, including tenure, are intrinsic components of the university. Accountability to a service or governmental organization can entail pressure to conform to the larger organizational context in ways that might compromise a scientist's ability to speak truth to power. Without a tradition of respecting an individual's rights to write and speak freely, and without a faculty association to represent those rights, there is a risk that corporations may silence legitimate dissent and critical research that runs counter to their official policies or that might be embarrassing. New understanding and means of negotiating must be devised in the absence of traditional academic protections. As long as there are enlightened leaders who are sympathetic to the scientific enterprise, alternative mechanisms will likely be sufficient, but lack the stability and strength of university policies. For example, when the chair worked closely with the MOHLTC on a system integration project (Goering et al., 2003), my home institution was concerned that I had not considered its agenda to be named as the lead system integration organization for the province. I had to defend my need to remain focused on the needs of the system, rather than the needs of my own organization. I argued that the HSRCU had to be somewhat independent of CAMH if we were to provide advice based on evidence rather than politics. This was a hard sell, especially for senior management, who were convinced that promoting CAMH as a system leader was a natural conclusion to an issue that was of importance to the organization's future. In the end I was not censored or restricted from taking my more neutral stance, but only because the individuals I spoke to valued academic freedom. If it had been otherwise, I might have been put in a precarious position with no formal policies or groups to turn to for support.

Researchers' closer proximity to research users and an interactive model of knowledge use are key components of Mode 2 operations, wherever they are situated. Close proximity, however, can also create increased tensions regarding the balance of rigour and relevance that is inherent to applied health services research. Collaborative research projects funded by the government with policy-makers as partners often create dilemmas that require thoughtful response. Frenk (1992) suggests that the research environment's structure is critical. He calls for an integrated approach in which scientists play dual roles of partner and scholar rather than create sub-units with an applied and traditional focus. I attempted to follow his approach in the chair program with a policy that all projects should both solve problems and also contribute new knowledge. But there were times when these dual goals came into conflict within projects and the research unit. For example, one of the chair's MOHLTC-funded, multi-year, multi-site evaluation projects aimed to study the process of policy implementation. I conducted qualitative interviews with key decision-makers at all levels, including senior ministry officials. As I analysed data, it became clear from the transcripts that there was a fair amount of criticism from the field about how the process had unfolded. Interviews with senior officials provided a different story that in some ways contradicted perceptions from the field and explained their actions. As my team discussed how to represent these different perspectives, we had to confront the possible ways in which our thinking might have been influenced by the MOHLTC's role as a funding source – not only for this particular study, but also for the global budget of our home organization. Staying true to data and paying neither too much nor too little attention to MOHLTC officials' perspectives was a more complex undertaking because of our multifaceted relationship. We were able to share drafts of our report with all of the respondents and were very relieved to find that MOHLTC did not become defensive about the way it was portrayed, even though we reported many criticisms of it. Having the right partner helps when a research unit located within a service agency works on a regular basis with government funding sources.

A Non-University Setting and Particular Research Career Paths

It was not an accident that I began my career as a clinical specialist in nursing at the psychiatric hospital that preceded CAMH. I moved into a more academic role through teaching nursing and then returning to conduct research and later complete my PhD in an interdisciplinary program. All of these activities were grounded in a desire to improve the front-line delivery of services for those with mental illness. My training meant that I was not socialized into a particular theoretical or methodological orientation. In many ways, leading a Mode 2 research environment suited me, but that is insufficient to create a strong fundamental and applied evidence base for my work. I must also respect and value the skills and knowledge that others with disciplinary strengths have where I do not. Learning how to combine aspects of Mode 1 and Mode 2 research has been an essential component of creating an environment that attracts and retains excellent researchers who also want to make a difference.

The chair's program enabled me to redefine my academic activities in order to support and train a wide range of fellows and trainees. In this regard, I found that a co-supervision model achieved a number of objectives. When I shared responsibility for a graduate student or fellow with a scientist in my unit who was new to supervision, the student had access to two people who could provide assistance; the scientist had a mentor; and I had the ability to take on more students because the workload and responsibility were shared. This model proved satisfactory to the trainees and helped to quickly expand the program's capacity. In a similar manner, I shifted my authorship role so that I was no longer first author on most of my publications. I supported trainees and junior faculty as they did the writing, while I provided guidance and editorial assistance. This arrangement did not always save time, but it did seem appropriate given our relative positions in the academic ranks.

Conclusion

Given the current trend towards distributing knowledge production sites, it is likely that we will need continued discussion about how best to design these alternative environments. If universities are considered the inner city, then housing developments in the suburbs will continue to expand. Health services research units can be funded in various ways and based in various organizational locations, but the chair's program suggests there are several general principles that may apply across these variations.

Just as transportation planning is critical to housing development, new research and education site planning should maintain ties with the university environment. Without these connections, it will be difficult to continue to educate the next generation of researchers – an endeavour that is necessary to keep scientists engaged in the formal academic enterprise. It is also important for universities to include these alternative environments and cross-appointed faculty positions in their activities to prepare students for a range of different career options. Embedded research units need their scientists to have access to graduate students and participate in the dialogue that accompanies their theoretical education. Universities need to include pragmatic learning opportunities so that students can observe different role models and experience research conducted in close relationships with healthcare providers and policy-makers in their own milieu.

Mixed, longer-term financing of new developments is another principle that requires careful consideration. User-commissioned research and consulting is a valuable source of resources, as well as a means of keeping the work attuned to real problems and the needs of those who purchase services and investigations. However, complete reliance on this type of external funding would result in a completely Mode 2 operational structure. Core funding of researcher salaries is necessary to provide the freedom to explore more fundamental questions and to engage in investigator-driven, peer-funded research that will result in publications and grants. Without such work, not only is the credibility of the researchers and consultants at risk, but also, and more importantly, the interplay between applied and basic knowledge is lost. Longer-term funding tied to a mandate for increasing capacity and exchange and linkage activities worked well in my chair's program, and is one way for research funding agencies to shape the infrastructure and sustain the future for embedded research units.

REFERENCES

Chafe, R., & Dobrow, M. (2008). Health services researchers working within healthcare organizations: The intriguing sound of three hands clapping. *Health Policy (Amsterdam)*, 4(2), 46–58.

Canadian Health Services Research Foundation. (2006). The creative professional activity dossier. *Recognition,* issue 1. Retrieved in July 2009 from http://www.cfhi-fcass.ca/libraries/recognition_english/the_creative_professional_activity_dossier_%e2%80%93_how_one_university_department_weighs_knowledge_exchange_activities_in_its_promotion_decisions.sflb.ashx

Denis, J., Lehoux, P., & Champagne, F. (2004). A knowledge utilization perspective on fine-tuning dissemination and contextualizing knowledge. In L. Lemieux-Charles & F. Champagne (Eds.), *Using knowledge and evidence in health care: Multidisciplinary perspectives* (pp. 18–40). Toronto: University of Toronto Press.

Dewa, C., Butterill, D., Durbin, J., & Goering, P. (2004). No matter how you land: Challenges of a longitudinal multi-site evaluation. *Canadian Journal of Program Evaluation, 19*(3), 1–28.

Ferlie, E., & Wood, M. (2003). Novel mode of knowledge production? Producers and consumers in health services research. *Journal of Health Services Research & Policy, 8*(Suppl 2), 51–7. http://dx.doi.org/10.1258/135581903322405171 Medline:14596748

Frenk, J. (1992). Balancing relevance and excellence: Organizational responses to link research with decision making. *Social Science & Medicine, 35*(11), 1397–404. http://dx.doi.org/10.1016/0277-9536(92)90043-P Medline:1462179

Gibbons, M., Limoges, C., Nowotny, H., Schwartzman, S., Scott, P., & Trow, M. (1994). Introduction. In M. Gibbons, ... (Eds.), *The new production of knowledge: The dynamics of science and research in contemporary societies* (pp. 1–16). London: Sage.

Goering, P., Butterill, D., Jacobson, N., & Sturtevant, D. (2003). Linkage and exchange at the organizational level: A model of collaboration between research and policy. *Journal of Health Services Research & Policy, 8*(Suppl 2), 14–19. http://dx.doi.org/10.1258/135581903322405126 Medline:14596743

Jacobson, N., Butterill, D., & Goering, P. (2005). Consulting as a strategy for knowledge transfer. *The Milbank Quarterly, 83*(2), 299–321. http://dx.doi.org/10.1111/j.1468-0009.2005.00348.x Medline:15960773

Jacobson, N., Butterill, D., & Goering, P. (2004). Organizational factors that influence university-based researchers' engagement in knowledge transfer activities. *Science Communication, 25*(3), 246–59. http://dx.doi.org/10.1177/1075547003262038

Jacobson, N., & Goering, P. (2006). Credibility and credibility work in knowledge transfer. *Policy Press, 2*(2), 151–65.

Landry, R. (2007). Commentary: Complementary perspectives on "speaking at cross-purposes or across boundaries." *Health Policy (Amsterdam), 3*(1), 40–3. Medline:19305754

Lomas, J. (2007). The in-between world of knowledge brokering. *BMJ, 334*(7585), 129–32. http://dx.doi.org/10.1136/bmj.39038.593380.AE Medline:17235094

Mitton, C., & Bate, A. (2007). Où sont les chercheurs? Speaking at cross-purposes or across boundaries? *Health Policy (Amsterdam), 3*(1), 32–7. Medline:19305752

Wasylenki, D.A., & Goering, P.N. (1995). The role of research in systems reform. *Canadian Journal of Psychiatry, 40*(5), 247–51. Medline:7553543

PART FIVE

Conclusion

13 Lessons Learned from the Chairs Program: An Inductive, Interpretive Analysis

LESLEY DEGNER

I vividly remember the morning after the federal budget announcement of 1998, when then-Finance Minister Paul Martin had unveiled the nursing research fund. I was walking into my research "home" at the St Boniface Research Centre and as I proceeded across the atrium and through the various areas en route to my office, several of my basic science colleagues stopped me. Their questions were essentially the same: "Lesley, are you going to get some of that money?" I replied, "Well, I am certainly going to try my best!" With the help of the faculty of nursing at the University of Manitoba, and with the support of central administration, we put an application forward that resulted in my chair being funded. This has led me into a ten-year adventure with my colleagues and the other chair holders, and along the way we have all learned some important lessons. My task in this chapter is to bring these lessons together in a form that might be useful for others who want to fund or participate in a similar adventure.

The identification of the themes I elaborate here emerged from a series of conversations at two successive chairs meetings in the fall of 2008 and spring of 2009. As the chairs presented and discussed each next-to-final chapter of this book, we identified common themes through a "committee of the whole" process of constant comparative analysis. This process was not dissimilar to what most qualitative analysts use in coding their field notes or interview data. However, ultimately, I have made an independent interpretation of the themes that emerged, so that any slippage that results from my more detached views of the contents of these chapters and our discussions is my responsibility alone.

The first time the chairs met in October 2000, we sat high in a conference room overlooking Parliament Hill. We could see the long meandering lines of Canadians waiting to pay their respects to the former prime minister, Pierre Elliot Trudeau, who had died earlier that week. In the intervening time the world has changed, and we have changed as well. What follows is an attempt to capture our evolution in response to a unique opportunity in Canadian healthcare and academia that we were privileged to access.

The Importance of Stable Funding

Most career awards in Canada provide for five to seven years of funding, which can be renewed at least once in some cases (such as the Canada Research chairs) and are not renewable in others (such as the previous National Cancer Institute of Canada Research Scientist awards). As CHSRF/CIHR chairs, we had the unique opportunity of a ten-year period in which to develop our programs, subject to a midterm review of our progress towards our goals. We also had the luxury of being able to design very individual and unique programs that would extend our research platforms and integrate graduate students and others into our research enterprise in new and meaningful ways. The ten-year time frame allowed for co-production of knowledge from practice, with our students and decision-making partners, in a way that would not have been possible within a shorter, more traditional period.

The chairs were all mid-career scientists – that is, we had established track records – and so we were able to take the risks demanded by an innovative program that required participants to be able to think about their research and their previous approaches to graduate training in new ways. Scholars who had yet to establish themselves and pass through the rites of tenure and promotion perhaps would not have been wise to take up such an enterprise, even had it been offered. Because of the long potential time frame that would be required to produce the "products" (grants and publications) traditionally valued in academia, in this alternative model of engaged scholarship with a variety of actors someone early in their career might place their future at risk by taking this approach. One wonders even today whether it is wise to encourage new assistant professors to work with decision-making partners to develop research programs, knowing the time such tasks will take and given the current publication requirements to achieve tenure and promotion in academia.

The Evolving Relationship with CHSRF

While we were all initially delighted to receive these awards (one of my colleagues likened them to the "academy awards" of nursing research), it quickly became apparent that reporting requirements for our yearly activities would be quite different from those attached to other such career funding. For example, in my previous career award I had not been required to submit even a final report, much less annual ones. Instead, common practice held that your productivity would be judged when you went forward for renewal of your funding. This way to provide funding had been prevalent for decades. There was an implicit trust in the ability of the peer-review process to identify and reward high performers. Those of us who had held such awards in the past were certainly in for a surprise with the chairs program's reporting requirements.

The time had come in Canada when concern over the responsible expenditure of government monies had gained significant momentum, and all agencies were required to actively demonstrate their stewardship of the funds they had been entrusted to disburse. It was in this atmosphere, in the early years of the new century, that the reporting requirements for the chairs evolved. However, such an evolution meant that new forms and templates had to be developed for this particular enterprise in the recently created CHSRF. The chairs and the budget departments of their universities received these new forms, which were new and mostly unfamiliar. As a result, there was a learning curve for the new reporting requirements, which caused frequent and sometimes frustrating delays for the chairs in trying to meet the budget deadlines and for CHSRF staff who were trying to do their work. Complicating this issue was the fact that the chairs' reports were required on a different time frame (calendar year) than is customary within the university (fiscal year), such that staffing within their budget departments was not particularly organized to meet the off-cycle deadline dates.

Beyond the budgetary reporting was the need for the chairs to complete two other annual tasks: reporting on their students and others involved in their chair programs (e.g., junior faculty, international visitors); and providing an annual report on their own activities. While on the face of it these seem to be straightforward exercises, they proved not to be. In an era of concern about disclosure of personal information, we had to seek annual permission from our students to include them in our databases. Templates for the annual chair reports evolved over time, which made it difficult to efficiently accumulate the "evidence" of productivity and effectiveness on an ongoing basis during the year. Many of us recognized early on that we would have to allocate at least some of our funding to hiring an individual to coordinate various administrative tasks if we, as the chairs, were to accomplish our primary mission.

Feedback on our annual reports was sometimes received with mixed feelings by the chairs. We were used to peer review, whereas our administrative reviews were sometimes different in flavour. In the early days of the chair program, these reviews were partly performed by individuals who had little experience with academic life. There seemed to be a fear that we would somehow "revert" to our old ways of isolation in our offices or labs, remote from our graduate students and decision-makers. In fact, we had been selected exactly because we did not practice our science in this way, and because we were all recognized for excellence in teaching. It took time for everyone to recognize that, given that the aim of the program was to increase evidence-informed practice and decision-making in the health system, research was the relevant platform for teaching and mentorship; the latter two simply do not, and cannot, occur in a science-free vacuum. Indeed, had we not maintained our credibility as scientists by obtaining research grants and producing publications, our future students would have been in jeopardy at the end of our chair program. It is a fact that students' funding is largely dependent on the research track record of their supervisors. Given Landry's findings (Chapter 3) that increasing teaching activities comes at the expense of decreasing publication outputs, it is not surprising that Armstrong (Chapter 10) writes in detail about issues related to time pressures for the chairs in this program.

Another issue was the accountability framework that each chair was asked to produce as a template for evaluating our programs. Each of us developed these in our own way, but there was tension between the administrative and academic views of what these frameworks should comprise. A rather amusing interchange occurred at my own midterm review when one CHSRF-appointed reviewer said, "But Lesley, this really isn't an accountability framework." I indicated that it might not be from an administrative perspective, but it was certainly helping me meet my program objectives. I added that at times I sensed that the program expected me to turn into an administrator, which was a lost cause, because I am a career scientist and intend to remain one! Laughter ensued, at least from some quarters, and we went on from there.

As it turns out, this concept of accountability frameworks as necessary to produce results was largely abandoned towards the end of the chairs program. It was gradually realized that the real program's outcomes (as opposed to pieces of paper with some process diagrams) emanate from people who pursue their creative work in a supportive environment. As Denis politely notes in Chapter 11, "We do not govern the chair." Armstrong provided a detailed analysis of this issue in Chapter 10; her observation that academics are not so much ungoverned as ungovernable, and the reasons for this, should be required reading for any funding agency considering an initiative similar to this one. What seemed to work best for most of us was having access to the collective wisdom of a hand-picked advisory committee to guide us through difficult decisions about the strategic directions for our programs. Several of these advisory committee structures are described in this book and could provide direction for other chairs tasked with similar objectives.

Pursuing Mode 2 Science

Reorienting our research such that it was now largely conducted through the lens of engaged scholarship was not novel for many of the chairs, but was for some such as myself, who had been studying underlying mechanisms in the psychosocial aspects of cancer for more than two decades. Some of the most interesting conversations we had as chairs were focused on our research, which was evolving within naturalistic environments in and around the healthcare system. These discussions were greatly enhanced by the diverse disciplinary backgrounds of the chairs; it was particularly useful for those of us from practice backgrounds such as nursing to interact with career social scientists. Their theoretical orientations in some ways collided with our more pragmatic approaches, but did so in a very creative way that enhanced the evolution of our programs.

Many of these innovative approaches stretched what at least some of us had considered appropriate scientific work at the outset of the program. With the chairs program, we had a unique opportunity to establish and maintain ongoing relationships with particular healthcare agencies and evolve our research within those environments over a ten-year period. The challenge was formidable, and there was always the chance that we might lose sight of our scientific autonomy, but the results of these experiments in Mode 2 science described by my colleagues speak for themselves. Clearly, these outcomes would not have happened in a shorter time span; even within a five-year time frame, one year is spent gearing up and the last one winding down, so the actual work of the project has to be compressed into the middle.

Goering raises an important point when she notes that her own program illustrated a combination of Mode 1 and Mode 2 science. Certainly one must have robust evidence to justify moving it into practice. In research conducted as part of his chair program, Landry found that knowledge transfer increased along with a university researcher's number of publications. Even though the focus in the chairs program was on co-production of knowledge with healthcare decision-makers, many of us continued to practice as Mode 1 scientists while extending our work into this relatively new model. Given Landry's findings, it is probably wise that we did. An important question remains: would we have had the credibility to work with decision-makers in these new scientific roles in the absence of this previous track record in more classic Mode 1 knowledge production indicators? Probably not. But DiCenso's description of engaged scholarship raises the always-important point that dissemination is irrelevant if research asks and answers the wrong question. Sketris notes the tension involved in maintaining depth in our own research field while engaging in Mode 2 science, which at least some of the chairs experienced.

One issue, discussed at some length, was the turnover of decision-makers during the course of our projects. The magnitude of this turnover was quite surprising to us as academics, since we are used to working with selected colleagues over decades. But we came to realize that this is just the way it is when working with people by virtue of their positions in organizations, as opposed to individual professors who have a career specializing in a particular field of research. We were on a learning curve here, and often our fears that a project would come to an end because a key individual in the organization was replaced were unfounded. Projects that are high priority within an organization usually remain high priority even with changing actors, which is a good thing given the considerable investment we, in our scientific roles, had made to these projects. Most of us learned how important the social marketing of our projects was, and we have all certainly expanded our skills in this regard.

Another issue we struggled with was the language in the field of – what should we call it? – knowledge transfer, knowledge translation, knowledge exchange, evidence-informed decision-making, engaged scholarship, and the list goes on. Even in our last meetings we could come to no clear consensus on the terminology, which speaks volumes. It is not surprising that colleagues from a variety of disciplines had this disconnect, but this was evident even within particular disciplines (such as nursing), indicating the scope of the dilemma of nomenclature. Part of this divergence was a result of the different theoretical frameworks we used to guide our individual programs. Perhaps the reality is that the terminology will continue to unfold and evolve as this field matures; it is clearly early days yet.

Our Graduate Students

Would we have worked in a similar fashion with graduate students without the funding provided by the chairs program? In some ways, yes, and in others, probably not. We were all experienced graduate supervisors, and in fact our perceived skill as such was one major criterion in the initial merit review. The major advantage within the program was that we had more flexible funding for our students; as a result, they could study full time, and we could recruit and select those who had the best potential to realize the objectives of our respective programs. The chairs program also allowed us to compare our mentorship styles. (For example, O'Brien-Pallas illustrates her mentorship style in Chapter 6.) This was facilitated by a specially planned mentorship workshop early in the chair program, which allowed us to externalize our approaches and consider them in light of what we were hearing from a mentorship expert. This type of opportunity rarely occurs in the usual course of academic life. At this workshop, we were all able to compare and contrast our styles and so learn from each other.

Perhaps the most exciting aspect of working with graduate students was the innovative programming that we were able to develop and subsequently offer. There are several excellent examples described in this book: Edwards' three-month research internship to complement graduate training and to help fast-track the research careers of nurses by improving their grantsmanship, publication, and knowledge translation skills (Chapter 7); Sketris' four-month residency program in drug use and policy that links graduate students and university researchers with decision-makers engaged in pharmaceutical policy development and program management (Chapter 8); Coyte's involvement of his students in generating financial data that was used to facilitate interaction between the Ontario Superior Court's role in interpreting the Canadian

Charter of Rights as opposed to the legislative goals of elected politicians (Chapter 4); and O'Brien-Pallas' six-month research apprenticeship for health service administrators, policy-makers, and nurses who wished to develop research skills related to planning health human resources (Chapter 6).

Graduate students would not have been offered these experiences and programs as part of regular academic programming, and in many cases they had the opportunity to interact with policy-makers, which rarely if ever happens during graduate degree course work. We expect that these experiences, facilitated by the chairs' funding, provided our graduates with career opportunities they might otherwise not have had. In fact, many of our graduates were lured into the practice and/or policy arena after completion of their master's degrees (hopefully for the benefit of our healthcare system), when we might have hoped to see them proceed to doctoral studies.

Another point that needs to be highlighted is the financial incentives that the chairs program allowed us to offer students. While these included the usual doctoral and postdoctoral fellowships, some of us paid our students' tuition as an incentive to study full-time and therefore graduate in a timely manner. As I said to potential students coming in to discuss our program, "This is a time-limited offer, so take advantage of it!" Another exciting aspect of our funding was the opportunity to take students with us to pivotal conferences that we judged to be good learning environments. The students were able to hear the leaders in the field present, and to actually see (and often talk with) the people whose work they had been reading. The inspirational impact of these experiences cannot be underestimated.

Our students also had opportunities to meet with students from regional training programs at specific joint meetings of the CADRE program, and with students from CIHR funded strategic training initiatives. These were fun and stimulating events that could be a bit overwhelming because of their intensity. There was significant cross-fertilization of ideas and experiences when students from different universities and disciplines talked with each other about their research and aspirations. We know that such singularly vivid events can leave lasting impressions that shape careers.

We are pleased to note that a process of formal and informal networking has emerged among our graduate students. They became ambassadors for our programs (see Edwards' Chapter 7) and in many cases led us to further innovation. This multiplication of ideas as a result of our interaction with graduate students is certainly not unique to the chairs program, but given the time and emphasis we had for such efforts, the possibility of this type of scaling up was there. We are indebted to our students for their vision and enthusiasm to determine how the unique educational experiences that we were trying to provide had benefited them, and in turn could benefit others. These informal networks were facilitated in no small part by the funding that allowed us to bring students from diverse geographic areas to visit or work in our programs.

International connections played an important role within these evolving academic programs. Although, at first, CHSRF staff seemed reluctant to consider how funding these international initiatives would contribute to capacity building in Canada, they gradually realized the reality of a global economy that is shaping science and academia more forcefully than ever before. Scientists can move easily and do their science anywhere that they are wanted, needed, and, in particular, supported. Our students have served as international ambassadors, and we are grateful to them for their commitment to and understanding of the importance of their role in this regard.

The Chairs

Although the individual chairs did not represent risk capital for this funding program, the program as a whole was obviously somewhat risky. This is probably what led to the unease among CHSRF staff members at the beginning of the program; they had funded us, but probably had some sense that the program could quickly become less than they hoped for. As chairs, I believe we were somewhat oblivious to these concerns, perhaps because we each knew our own work ethic and our compulsive drive to succeed at anything we take on. These are issues that, in retrospect, we could have and should have addressed explicitly at the onset of the program to avoid some of the unconstructive communication that occurred between CHSRF staff and the chairs during that time.

One of the most salient features of the program was that the chairs were brought together twice annually. We all agree that this was a fundamentally important aspect of the chairs program, even though at times it seemed a bit of a burden in light of our other ever-expanding responsibilities. Tackling any major enterprise as a group is dramatically different than doing so alone. The private consultations that occurred at these meetings between and among chairs were critical; as one chair noted, it helped to know that you were not crazy if you were having a certain problem. Interestingly, we had very little time on our own in the first few years – the agendas were packed with administrative items, and we had to specifically request and indeed push for such private meeting times. We have noted that some recent funding programs for mid-career scientists through the national funding councils do not provide a mechanism for scientists to meet together regularly during their career awards, and we view this as a lost opportunity.

The chairs have played an important role in mentoring doctoral and postdoctoral students who have since transitioned into junior faculty positions. This more immediate renewal of the professoriate is one outcome of the chairs program that is already in place and reaping benefits. Some of these individuals are already successful scientists with their own national career awards and operating grants. It was important for us as individuals to see these outcomes before the end of the chair program to ensure that at least part of our legacy was in place while the rest matured.

Lessons Learned

So what do we really know as a result of this experiment? We were all charged with the task of bringing knowledge to practice in our various fields, so the least we can do for people coming after us who might be interested in a similar experiment is to acknowledge what we think we have learned. These are the lessons that I think my colleagues have elucidated:

- A longer time frame than most career awards (ten years versus five or seven) is required if you are truly going to pursue Mode 2 science; that is, the co-production of knowledge with decision-makers.
- Clear communication between chairs and the funding agency regarding the role of scientific work is also required; that is, Mode 1 science is essential to maintaining credibility while engaging in Mode 2 science.
- Graduate training can be greatly enhanced by providing new experiences to engage with decision-maker partners in practice, but those decision-makers may be so impressed by the students that they entice them away from academia.

- Accountability mechanisms must be sensible and designed to facilitate rather than impede obtaining the desired results of the program.
- Designing a program with a wide disciplinary mix of academics who meet together on a regular basis can yield unexpected dividends.
- International initiatives provide enriching experiences for graduate students and can stimulate innovative approaches to service delivery in healthcare.

While there are many other lessons that could be listed, these are the most salient for those designing such a program. More specific lessons on the process of actualizing the work can be found in this book's individual chapters, and these would be of particular interest for academics with similar disciplinary orientations who are trying to accomplish the research, mentoring, and knowledge exchange mission that was our goal.

Conclusion

One of the things I note in the chapters here is the modesty of my colleagues with respect to the intellectual contributions that they have made to the success of the chairs program over the past decade. A program is only as good as its people and their ideas. The creativity of the individual chair programs is clearly evident in these chapters, and is the product of the clear thinking and perseverance of a group of exceptional Canadian academics. We are in their debt when we consider the number of graduate students they have mentored over the past decade. These students are the future academics and scientists who will, in turn, guide their own graduate students in the ensuing years. If we consider the reach of the chairs program in terms of the number of person years of graduate student advisement that will occur over the next generation as a result, it is really quite astounding. I remember when we asked Jonathan Lomas at our first meeting how many students he thought we should each take into our programs and graduate before the end of the chair program. He very wisely responded, "More than one." I trust he is pleased with the results of the program.

We can only hope that our academic children and grandchildren will come of age in an era where there is sufficient grant money for them to conduct their science through the model of engaged scholarship we have described in this book. This is an issue that always troubles professors; you ask students to spend many years studying with you, knowing that access to grant funding rises and falls according to the prevalent political ideologies. We never know what that environment will be like when our students graduate. But if the Canadian healthcare system is to become truly evidence-informed, then we all need to be sure that these young scientists will get the resources they need to work effectively. Otherwise, our efforts may well have been in vain.

Contributors

Nabil Amara is an associate professor in the Department of Management of the Faculty of Business at Laval University in Quebec City. He was also the co-director of the CHSRF/CIHR Chair in Knowledge Transfer and Innovation at Laval University. His most significant works on innovation and knowledge transfer have been published in *Research Policy, Public Administration Review, Science Communication, Technological Forecasting and Social Change,* and *Technovation.*

Pat Armstrong is a professor in the Department of Sociology at York University and is the author or co-author of more than a dozen books. She also served as a CHSRF/CIHR Chair in Applied Health Services and Nursing Research.

Patricia Conrad joined CHSRF in 2005 as the director of the CADRE program and subsequently became the chief of policy and planning with the Nova Scotia Department of Health. She worked with Dr Ingrid Sketris, one of CHSRF's research chairs, to implement the Drug Use Management and Policy Research Residency. She coordinated the funding proposal for the Atlantic Regional Training Centre – a joint initiative involving Dalhousie University, Memorial University, the University of New Brunswick, and the University of PEI that was funded by CHSRF. She is currently the executive director of policy, planning, and intergovernmental affairs with the Nova Scotia Department of Health.

Peter C. Coyte is a professor of health economics in the Institute of Health Policy, Management, and Evaluation in the Faculty of Medicine at the University of Toronto, and was a CHSRF/CIHR Chair in Health

Care Settings and Canadians. He has been recognized for his scholarly contributions through receipt of a CIHR Senior Investigator Award, a Kappa Delta Award from the American Academy of Orthopaedic Surgeons, and a Young Investigator Award from the Association of University Programs in Health Administration.

Lesley Degner is a professor in the Faculty of Nursing and an associate professor in the Department of Family Medicine at the University of Manitoba. She was recently appointed a foreign adjunct professor in the Department of Nursing at the Karolinska Institute in Stockholm. Dr Degner held the CHSRF/CIHR Chair in Nursing Care focused on the development of evidence-based nursing practice in cancer care, palliative care, and cancer prevention. She also serves as a consultant in evidence-based nursing practice at the Health Sciences Centre in Winnipeg.

Jean-Louis Denis is a full professor in the Department of Health Administration and a researcher with the Groupe de recherche interdisciplinaire en santé in the Faculty of Medicine at the University of Montreal. He held the CHSRF/CIHR Chair in the Transformation and Governance of Health Care Organizations. Dr Denis is a member of the Royal Society of Canada and is the academic coordinator of the EXTRA program, an initiative that teaches executives about the use of research-based evidence in healthcare organizations.

Alba DiCenso held the CHSRF/CIHR Chair in Advanced Practice Nursing at McMaster University, where she is a professor of nursing and of clinical epidemiology and biostatistics, and the director of the CHSRF/CIHR Ontario Training Centre in Health Services and Policy Research. An exemplary educator, researcher, and author, she is internationally known for her pioneering work in evidence-based nursing and is an expert on advanced practice nursing, including the roles and effectiveness of nurse practitioners and clinical nurse specialists in Canada. She has influenced policy on the development of nurse practitioners and their place in healthcare systems at the provincial, national, and international levels.

Nancy Edwards is a professor of nursing and of epidemiology and community medicine at the University of Ottawa, and is a world-class scholar in the design and conduct of multi-level and multi-strategy community health programs. She held a CHSRF/CIHR Nursing Research

Chair and is scientific director of CIHR's Population and Public Health Institute. Her awards include the University of Ottawa 2006 Award of Excellence in Research and the Tianjin Haihe Award from the Tianjin Municipal Government in China for outstanding contributions to their university. In 2006, the City of Ottawa proclaimed "Nancy Edwards Day" in recognition of her many contributions to the health of her city and country.

Paula Goering is a professor of psychiatry in the University of Toronto Faculty of Medicine and is cross-appointed to the Faculty of Nursing, Institute of Medical Science, and the Department of Health Policy, Management, and Evaluation. She held a CHSRF/CIHR Health Services Chair. In her role as the director of the Health Systems Research and Consulting Unit at the Centre for Addiction and Mental Health, Goering has overseen a wide range of applied research activities that include synthesizing existing scientific information for policy and planning use, designing and conducting investigations for specific providers and planners, and educating stakeholders.

Laureen Hayes is currently a research officer in the Nursing Health Services Research Unit and the University of Toronto. From 2006 to 2010, she was the research associate for the CHSRF/CIHR Chair in Nursing Health Human Resources. Hayes contributed to the work of the chair through her involvement in several studies in all stages of the research process, liaison with stakeholders and chair participants, ongoing communication with the chair advisory committee, and facilitation of knowledge transfer activities.

Lise Lamothe is a professor in the Department of Health Administration and a regular researcher at Public Health Research Institute at the University of Montreal. Her research interests include governance and the professional dynamics associated with the transformation of healthcare organizations, notably the challenges raised by multimorbidity. She is also interested in the issues that surround institutional mergers, the formation of networks of integrated services, and the structuring effects of NCIT in the transformation of clinical work processes. She is a member of the board of l'Hôpital du Sacré-Coeur de Montréal.

Réjean Landry was the holder of a CHSRF/CIHR Chair in Knowledge Transfer and Innovation. Dr Landry is a professor in the Department of

Management of the Faculty of Business at Laval University in Quebec City, where he teaches on knowledge transfer and knowledge management. He has published many quantitative papers on knowledge transfer and innovation.

Erin (Morrison) Leith is the senior advisor for collaboration for innovation and improvement at the Canadian Foundation for Healthcare Improvement in Ottawa, Ontario. Currently, she manages several of CFHI's regional partnerships for health system improvement, including a Northwest Territories partnership to improve and integrate the delivery of chronic disease management services. In 2010, Leith led the design and delivery of the national Picking up the Pace conference, which showcased primary healthcare innovations from across Canada and abroad and was lead of the CADRE program. She has a background in nursing and health administration, and prior to joining CFHI worked as a registered nurse with the Capital District Health Authority in Halifax, Nova Scotia.

Jonathan Lomas was the founding head of CHSRF for ten years. His career – including fifteen years as a professor and five years as the head of the Centre for Health Economics and Policy Analysis at McMaster University – focuses on the spread of research and innovation to health systems decision-making. Among his many awards, he has a Doctorat Honoris Causa from the University of Montreal, is a specially elected Fellow of the Royal Society of Canada, and has been appointed an Officer of the Order of Canada.

Anne McManus was the coordinator of the Transformation and Governance of Health Organizations Chair at the University of Montreal.

Linda O'Brien-Pallas is a professor in the Faculties of Nursing and Medicine at the University of Toronto and the director and co-principal investigator of the Nursing Health Services Research Unit (University of Toronto site). Recognized as a world authority on nursing human resources, she held the inaugural CHSRF/CIHR Chair in Nursing/Health Human Resources and is a fellow of the Canadian Academy of Health Sciences.

Louise Potvin is a professor in the Department of Social and Preventive Medicine, is a researcher with GRIS (an interdisciplinary health research group), and has served as a CHSRF/CIHR Chair in Community Approaches and Health Inequalities at the University of Montreal.

Ingrid S. Sketris is a professor of pharmacy at Dalhousie University. She was the president of the Association of Faculties of Pharmacy of Canada and is a fellow of the Canadian Society of Hospital Pharmacists and the American College of Clinical Pharmacy. She held the CHSRF/CIHR Chair in Capacity for Applied Developmental Research and Evaluation in Health Services. Her research involves examining approaches to increase the uptake of evidence-based drug therapies and the effectiveness of policy levers used by pharmacare programs to provide effective and affordable drugs.

FSC
www.fsc.org
MIX
Papier | Fördert
gute Waldnutzung
FSC® C083411

Zeitfracht Medien GmbH
Ferdinand-Jühlke-Straße 7
99095 Erfurt, Deutschland
produktsicherheit@kolibri360.de